THE NATIONAL ACADEMIES

National Academy of Sciences
National Academy of Engineering
Institute of Medicine
National Research Council

The **National Academy of Sciences** is a private, nonprofit, self-perpetuating society of distinguished scholars engaged in scientific and engineering research, dedicated to the furtherance of science and technology and to their use for the general welfare. Upon the authority of the charter granted to it by the Congress in 1863, the Academy has a mandate that requires it to advise the federal government on scientific and technical matters. Dr. Bruce M. Alberts is president of the National Academy of Sciences.

The **National Academy of Engineering** was established in 1964, under the charter of the National Academy of Sciences, as a parallel organization of outstanding engineers. It is autonomous in its administration and in the selection of its members, sharing with the National Academy of Sciences the responsibility for advising the federal government. The National Academy of Engineering also sponsors engineering programs aimed at meeting national needs, encourages education and research, and recognizes the superior achievements of engineers. Dr. Wm. A. Wulf is president of the National Academy of Engineering.

The **Institute of Medicine** was established in 1970 by the National Academy of Sciences to secure the services of eminent members of appropriate professions in the examination of policy matters pertaining to the health of the public. The Institute acts under the responsibility given to the National Academy of Sciences by its congressional charter to be an adviser to the federal government and, upon its own initiative, to identify issues of medical care, research, and education. Dr. Kenneth I. Shine is president of the Institute of Medicine.

The **National Research Council** was organized by the National Academy of Sciences in 1916 to associate the broad community of science and technology with the Academy's purposes of furthering knowledge and advising the federal government. Functioning in accordance with general policies determined by the Academy, the Council has become the principal operating agency of both the National Academy of Sciences and the National Academy of Engineering in providing services to the government, the public, and the scientific and engineering communities. The Council is administered jointly by both Academies and the Institute of Medicine. Dr. Bruce M. Alberts and Dr. Wm. A. Wulf are chairman and vice chairman, respectively, of the National Research Council.

ADOLESCENT RISK AND VULNERABILITY

CONCEPTS AND MEASUREMENT

Baruch Fischhoff, Elena O. Nightingale, Joah G. Iannotta, *Editors*

Board on Children, Youth, and Families

Division of Behavioral and Social Sciences and Education

National Research Council

and

Institute of Medicine

NATIONAL ACADEMY PRESS
Washington, D.C.

NATIONAL ACADEMY PRESS 2101 Constitution Avenue, N.W. Washington, D.C. 20418

NOTICE: The project that is the subject of this report was approved by the Governing Board of the National Research Council, whose members are drawn from the councils of the National Academy of Sciences, the National Academy of Engineering, and the Institute of Medicine. The members of the committee responsible for the report were chosen for their special competences and with regard for appropriate balance.

The study was supported by Grant No. B7128 and B6815 between the National Academy of Sciences and the Carnegie Corporation of New York. Any opinions, findings, conclusions, or recommendations expressed in this publication are those of the author(s) and do not necessarily reflect the views of the organizations or agencies that provided support for this project.

Library of Congress Cataloging-in-Publication Data

Adolescent risk and vulnerability : approaches to setting priorities to reduce their burden / Baruch Fischhoff, Elena O. Nightingale, Joah G. Iannotta, Editors.

p. cm.

Includes bibliographical references.

ISBN 0-309-07620-X (perfectbound)

1. Risk-taking in adolescence (Psychology)—United States—Congresses. 2. Teenagers—United States—Social conditions—Congresses. 3. Teenagers—Health risk assessment—United States—Congresses. 4. Youth—Government policy—United States—Congresses. I. Fischhoff, Baruch, 1946- II. Nightingale, Elena O. III. Iannotta, Joah G.

HV1431 .A633 2001

362.7'083'0973—dc21

2001005256

Additional copies of this report are available from the National Academy Press, 2101 Constitution Avenue, N.W., Lock Box 285, Washington, D.C. 20055.

Call (800) 624-6242 or (202) 334-3313 (in the Washington metropolitan area)

This report is also available online at http://www.nap.edu

Printed in the United States of America

Suggested citation: National Research Council and Institute of Medicine. (2001). *Adolescent risk and vulnerability: Concepts amd measurement.* Board on Children, Youth, and Families. Division of Behavioral and Social Sciences and Education. Baruch Fischhoff, Elena O. Nightingale, and Joah G. Iannotta, Eds. Washington, DC: National Academy Press.

ELEANOR E. MACCOBY *(Liaison, Division of Behavioral and Social Sciences and Education)*, Department of Psychology (Emerita, Stanford University

WILLIAM ROPER *(Liaison, Institute of Medicine),* School of Public Health, University of North Carolina, Chapel Hill

Elena O. Nightingale, *Scholar-in-Residence*

Michele D. Kipke, *Director*

Mary Graham, *Associate Director, Dissemination and Communications*

Sonja Wolfe, *Administrative Associate*

Joah G. Iannotta, *Research Assistant*

Contents

Preface

In September 1997 the Board on Children, Youth, and Families organized a planning meeting on indicators for the safety and security of adolescents. A number of important ideas developed in this workshop, including the need to reassess and redefine adolescent vulnerability in order to develop more effective policies and programmatic interventions to safeguard young people.

Early in 2000, and under the auspices of the Board, the two moderators in the planning meeting, Elena Nightingale, Scholar-in-Residence with the Board on Children, Youth, and Families, and Baruch Fischhoff, Professor of Social and Decision Sciences at Carnegie Mellon University, initiated the development of a workshop to stimulate thinking about the meaning of adolescent vulnerability, the methodologies that can be employed to measure vulnerability and its disparate predisposing risk factors, and the steps that would advance the work necessary for setting priorities for policies and practices to reduce the total burden of vulnerability for young people.

A small planning group was formed to develop a workshop on reconceptualizing adolescent risk and vulnerability. This committee included Robert William Blum, Professor of Pediatrics at the University of Minnesota; Martha R. Burt, Program Director and Principal Research Associate at the Urban Institute; Susan G. Millstein, Professor of Pediatrics at the University of California at San Francisco; as well as Baruch Fischhoff and Elena O. Nightingale, who served as co-chairs of the group. The task was to plan a workshop that would bring together the work and experience of several disciplines, from health science to psychology, decision science, and economics, that could further current research and thinking about adolescent vulnerability. As a part of this task, Drs. Blum, Burt, Millstein, and Fischhoff and their colleagues wrote papers that focused on the particular aspect of reconceptualizing adolescent vulnerability within their respective field of expertise. These papers were deliberately interconnected with the intention of generating not only a new way of defining adolescent vulnerability, but also of creating new methodological approaches to conducting research on both vulnerability and positive attributes of young people that could offer a more effective knowledge base for policy and intervention than available currently.

With funding from Carnegie Corporation of New York, the *Workshop on Adolescent Risk and Vulnerability: Setting Priorities* took place on March 13, 2001, in Washington, DC. The workshop's goal was to put into perspective the total burden of vulnerability that adolescents face, taking advantage of the growing societal concern for adolescents, the need to set priorities for meeting adolescents' needs, and the opportunity to apply decision-making perspectives to this critical area. The workshop included five sessions, the first four of which were based on the papers prepared for the workshop.

The first session examined a new conceptual framework for understanding and moderating adolescent vulnerability. The second session focused on the social costs of adolescent risk taking and vulnerability. The discussion included ways to model the lifelong costs and benefits of risky behavior in adolescence and the payoffs of interventions to reduce them. The third session proposed ways to assess the total burden of adolescents' vulnerability and its components, as well as what indices are useful to monitor progress in reducing vulnerability and what social mechanisms can be used to set priorities for reducing them. The fourth session centered on perceptions of vulnerability by adolescents and by adults and how their accuracy can be measured and analyzed. How beliefs about risks influence risk taking and adolescents' ability to manage the risks and vulnerabilities they face also were discussed. The final session considered the implications of these approaches to adolescent vulnerability as well as opportunities they might provide to bridge research, policy, and practice.

This report includes an introduction by co-chairs Fischhoff and Nightingale that summarizes issues raised at the workshop and the four papers prepared and presented by the planning group members. The summary reflects the presentations and perspectives of the presenters and participants at the workshop. It is not intended to be a comprehensive review of all the issues that emerged at the workshop or of all those relevant to adolescent risk and vulnerability. Rather, it attempts to highlight key issues and viewpoints that emerged from the rich discussions that took place. The information distilled in this summary is drawn from the presentations of the speakers and the dialogue that ensued, and every effort has been made to accurately reflect the speakers' content and viewpoints.

The papers in this volume were reviewed in draft form by the workshop discussants, chosen for their diverse perspectives and technical expertise. For their insightful and constructive comments, we thank Mark Cohen, Susan Curnan, Peter Edelman, Beatrix A. Hamburg, Lloyd J. Kolbe, Richard M. Lerner, Ann S. Masten, Gary B. Melton, Shepherd Smith, Matthew Stagner, and Heather Weiss. We also especially thank Anne Petersen, who generously gave of her time to oversee the review and further strengthen the contents of this volume. Although the individuals listed provided constructive comments and suggestions, it must be emphasized that responsibility for the final content of the volume rests entirely with the authors.

The Board is particularly grateful to the planning group that developed the workshop framework and prepared the papers included in this volume. We especially thank Elena O. Nightingale and Baruch Fischhoff, who co-chaired the workshop and who, with Joah Iannotta, edited this volume, and Mary Graham, who provided assistance in coordinating this publication.

Michele D. Kipke, *Director*
Board on Children, Youth, and Families

1

Adolescent Risk and Vulnerability: Overview

Elena O. Nightingale and Baruch Fischhoff

INTRODUCTION

Adolescents obviously do not always act in ways that serve their own best interests, even as defined by them. Sometimes their perception of their own risks, even of survival to adulthood, is larger than the reality; in other cases, they underestimate the risks of particular actions or behaviors. It is possible, indeed likely, that some adolescents engage in risky behaviors because of a perception of invulnerability—the current conventional wisdom of adults' views of adolescent behavior. Others, however, take risks because they feel vulnerable to a point approaching hopelessness (Fischhoff et al., 2000). In either case, these perceptions can prompt adolescents to make poor decisions that can put them at risk and leave them vulnerable to physical or psychological harm that may have a negative impact on their long-term health and viability.

Despite the widespread view that adolescents feel personally invulnerable, both scientific evidence and direct discussions with them show that most have serious concerns, many of them based on real-life factors that present obstacles difficult for any individual—adult or minor—to overcome. Chronic diseases such as diabetes, cystic fibrosis, or asthma can pose daunting challenges and even panic. Young people feel threatened by violence, not knowing which minor incident or sideways glance will get out of control, or when they might be in the wrong place at the wrong time. Even if the economy is sound, many adolescents worry about having a decent and meaningful job or career. Racial relations and poverty are special concerns. These are some components of the burden of vulnerability perceived by adolescents in the United States, which might contribute to their participation in risky behaviors such as unsafe sexual activity, alcohol or drug intoxication, risky driving, and more (Fischhoff et al., 1998; Lindberg et al., 2000).

Assessing the Burden of Adolescent Vulnerability

Adolescents today face complex and changing environments in which many things can go right and wrong. If we are to serve and protect them, we must have a full appreciation of these environments as well as society's opportunities to shape them. Research that can conceptualize, measure, and evaluate the total burden of adolescent vulnerability is sorely needed. New research approaches must be designed to explore as comprehensively as possible the complexities of coexisting risk and protective factors in particular settings as well as variations in the ways adolescent perceive their own vulnerability. Without such knowledge, practitioners are in a poor position to design the best possible programs to facilitate healthy adolescent development and well-being, and policy makers lack the research-based information that can inform their decisions.

Previous approaches to risk taking in young people include a developmental psychosocial model (Levitt et al., 1991). This model encompasses three elements: knowledge about the risk, management skills to deal with it, and the personal meaning of the risk, all within a developmental perspective. The developmental changes in the personal meaning of risks are of particular relevance here.

In a recent review of research on programmatic investments in young people of various ages, Danziger and Waldfogel (2000) demonstrated that early childhood investments pay off for children as they develop. What is also clear from this volume is the need to invest in children as they get older, particularly during adolescence, in which young people experience multiple transitions such as new school environments and changing peer and family dynamics. This volume also documents the lack of systematic research on investments in adolescents that could support policy and practice that better meet the needs of youngsters 10 to 18 years of age.

Of central importance to filling this research gap is to reconceptualize approaches that could deal effectively with the complexity of adolescent vulnerabilities by capturing both the total burden of vulnerability of youth in general and of those youth with special problems, particularly chronic illness or extreme poverty. Both adolescents and adults need to know the actual burden of adolescents' vulnerability and be aware of each other's perceptions of such before policies and practices can be developed to reduce the burden. Knowing the size of the overall burden is essential in order to decide what personal and societal resources to devote to this problem relative to other priorities. Knowledge about the relative size of different problems and of opportunities for risk reduction is required so that investment in current interventions can be made for the "best buys" and so that better means can be devised to help adolescents. In sum, research that can provide knowledge about the relative burden of adolescent vulnerability could help to protect adolescents, assist practitioners in designing youth development programs, and support policy makers in setting priorities for allocating resources.

Once new approaches have been developed to capture the burden of adolescent vulnerability, additional knowledge can be gained by systematic study or experimentation. An important and accessible place to begin would be to mine existing data sets from the vulnerability perspective; this could lead to closing the gap between perceived and measured risks in the short term while new data are being collected. During the past decade, a growing number of cross-sectional and longitudinal data sets have addressed adolescent risk and sources of vulnerability that lend themselves to the proposed activity. For example, a new source of data that has the potential to significantly advance our knowledge base of behavioral development among adolescents is the National Longitudinal Study of Adolescent Health (Blum et al., 2000; Svetaz et al., 2000). From the collection of longitudinal data, it will be possible to examine how the timing and tempo of puberty influence social and cognitive development among teenagers. This data set permits analysts to examine how family-, school-, and individual-level risk and protective factors are associated with adolescent health and morbidity (e.g., emotional health, violence, substance use, and sexuality). Other longitudinal data sets that could be mined include the National Longitudinal Survey of Youth, the Children and Young Adults of the National Survey of Children and Youth, and the Program of Research on the Causes and Correlates of Delinquency: Denver Youth. Sources of cross-sectional research data that could be useful include the Youth Risk Behavior Surveillance Survey, Monitoring the Future, and the Survey of Children with Special Health Care Needs.

Creating a New Research Base

In response to the need for new research, the Board on Children, Youth, and Families formed an ad hoc planning committee to develop papers in conjunction with a workshop that would stimulate new thinking about adolescent risk and vulnerability. The papers and workshop sought to take a different approach to the high-risk behaviors of adolescents by defining and devising measurements for the burden of adolescent vulnerabilities, the interactions between risks and protective factors, total costs and benefits of interventions, evaluation of interventions, and how best to learn about different perceptions of risk by adolescents and adults. Authors also suggested when and how these new approaches could be applied to existing data sets and to designing new longitudinal and cross-sectional studies.

This volume describes the workshop, entitled *Adolescent Risk and Vulnerability: Setting Priorities,* which drew together experts with diverse scholarly and professional perspectives, ranging from health to economics, decision science, and psychology, in order to apply these multiple perspectives to improving the well-being and future prospects of adolescents in the United States. Each of the four papers presents a distinct approach to adolescent risk and vulnerability. They were prepared for, presented, and discussed at the workshop held at the National Academies on March 13, 2001.

In both the workshop and this volume, we hope to place adolescent vulnerability into perspective, taking advantage of the growing societal concern for adolescents, and the need to set priorities for investment of limited resources (Burt, 1998; Burt and Levy, 1987). With the best understanding that research allows, we can begin to assess how to intervene in the most effective and efficacious manner. The potential impact of research that can guide investments in adolescent development in both individuals and our society cannot be underestimated. Benefits may accrue even for those adolescents who do not experience a development program directly because peers who do participate become more focused and motivated in school, more engaged in their communities, and less involved in risk behaviors (Danziger and Waldfogel, 2000).

The workshop discussions served to bring the ideas in the papers together toward an integrated research approach for reducing adolescent vulnerability. The following provides brief summaries of the papers and the points made by discussants who reviewed each of them.

PAPER AND DISCUSSION SUMMARIES

Perceptions of Risk and Vulnerability, by Susan G. Millstein and Bonnie L. Halpern-Felsher, examines the beliefs underlying adolescents' decisions, with particular attention to how to evaluate their competence. They find that, contrary to popular belief, the scientific literature does not support the notion that adolescents view themselves as uniquely invulnerable to harm; rather, their perceptions of invulnerability resemble those of the adults around them. This myth can distort programs and policies for adolescents by suggesting a level of incompetence that warrants more manipulative interventions and fewer opportunities for exploration and growth. Indeed, in some ways, adolescents show a deep sense of vulnerability, as when asked about their overall chance of premature death (Fischoff et al., 2000).

The authors demonstrate the importance of adolescents' risk perceptions for developmental theory, programming, and setting standards of decision-making competence (e.g., for making health decisions). They also describe the methodological issues facing such studies. Many have used hypothetical situations, which allow standardization across subjects, but may seem unrealistic to many. Others have asked for judgments of ambiguous events (Fischhoff, 1996; Halpern-Felsher et al., 2001), or used verbal quantifiers as response modes (e.g., the use of "very likely," "likely"; for further discussion, see Biehl and Halpern-Felsher, 2001), making it difficult to evaluate the accuracy of the beliefs that are expressed. The paper makes the case for using more realistic situations in order to provide ecological validity. Doing so will make it easier to characterize the relationships between adolescent behaviors and the perceived risks and benefits of their actions. Those studies will have to consider the context within which adolescents evaluate their options. For example, if an adolescent does not believe that he or she will live beyond the age of 30, the risk of AIDS may have little influence on sexual behavior.

In their discussion of Millstein and Halpern-Felsher's paper, both Richard Lerner and Ann Masten noted its potential for guiding program and policy innovations that will promote positive youth development. They pointed to the paper's new and useful insights regarding how perceptions influence adolescents' decision making about risky behaviors. They suggested research into adolescents' perceptions relevant to improved decision making; developing an ecological perspective for understanding vulnerability; understanding (and combating) myths about adolescent vulnerability; and a continuing focus on positive youth development (Masten, 2001).

Vulnerability, Risk, and Protection, by Robert William Blum, Clea McNeely, and James Nonnemaker, presents a model for understanding the vulnerability of adolescents to undesirable outcomes, from the individual to the macro level. Using data from the National Longitudinal Study of Adolescent Health (Add Health), the authors applied the model to evaluating the effects of protective factors on risky behaviors, such as violence, cocaine use, and sexual intercourse. Meaningful interventions require understanding of the interactions and complexities of these processes. For example, school classroom management climate was proven to be a protective factor against weapon-related violence, but not against cocaine use. Effective policies and interventions must take into account the connections between vulnerability and protective processes.

Although the framework in the Blum et al. paper offers the possibility of identifying and reducing negative educational, social, and health outcomes that may mitigate several negative outcomes at once, and has potential for being quite productive, discussant Lloyd Kolbe was concerned that the complexity of the model might make it difficult to translate theory into practice. To take advantage of the strengths of the framework, he suggested using it to identify protective factors, relationships, and processes that seem particularly effective and enabling appropriate social institutions (e.g., public and private agencies, youth-serving organizations) to use underutilized protective factors in future interventions to help young people. Because the model demonstrates interaction of risk and protective factors in several areas, it could promote collaboration among educational, social service, and health agencies to reduce adolescent vulnerability and risk.

Kolbe identified future research opportunities, including articulating and measuring protective factors and monitoring them over time; and conducting longitudinal-cohort community-based studies, such as Healthy Passages,[1] of how variables evolve over time as well as intervention research

---

[1]Healthy Passages: A Community-based Longitudinal Study of Adolescent Health, supported by the Centers for Disease Control and Prevention (CDC), is scheduled to begin in June 2001 in three communities; Birmingham, Los Angeles, and Houston. CDC funds were awarded to three universities to conduct the research: University of Alabama at Birmingham (Michael Windle, Ph.D., Principal Investigator); University of California at Los Angeles/RAND (Mark Schuster, M.D., Ph.D., Principal Investigator); and University of Texas-Houston (Guy Parcel, Principal Investigator). Further information on the study is available from Project Officer Jo Anne Grunbaum, Ed.D., at jpg9@cdc.gov.

determining whether these variables can be modified. Kolbe noted both the difficulty and the importance of such synthetic research.

According to discussant Beatrix Hamburg, the model presented by Blum et al. has potential to deal with complex interactions among variables, macrolevel influences, and contextual specificity. What happens within a context (e.g., school), such as attendance or peer acceptance, contributes to the final outcome, even in a positive environment.

Among macrolevel variables, chronic disease is of special concern for the adolescent (Hamburg, 1982). A large and growing number of adolescents live with diseases such as cystic fibrosis, diabetes, asthma, and some cancers, all of which were once fatal at an early age. Now, due to medical advances, adolescents can live a long time with a disorder that can be treated but not cured. A disease and its treatment impose risks related to the developmental tasks of adolescence, such as establishing a positive body and self-image as well as peer acceptance, among other tasks. The specter of being permanently afflicted with damage and disability confers a substantial risk. As adolescents attempt to negotiate normative developmental tasks as well as demanding medical regimens, the risks imposed by chronic disease can lead to adverse outcomes in medical, emotional, social, and educational spheres. Parents often have little understanding or guidance in coping with these issues, and, at best, tend to become over-protective and anxious. Family conflict is common. For these reasons, adolescence is an especially vulnerable period for those with chronic illness. The Blum et al. model could help identify realistic approaches to reducing these risks and making best use of protective factors. The model also can be applied to data sources in addition to Add Health, among them Monitoring the Future and the Youth Risk Behavior Survey.

Modeling the Payoffs of Interventions to Reduce Adolescent Vulnerability, by Martha R. Burt, Janine M. Zweig, and John Roman, emphasizes that adolescents establish behavior patterns and activities such as smoking and sexual activity that affect their lifetime well-being. However, these long-term consequences can be ignored, leading to insufficient investment in adolescents, whose short-term morbidity and mortality are relatively low. Traditional methods for estimating costs of health risks and outcomes do not provide good assessments of all the costs and benefits—social, economic, and human. The paper presents models for estimating the full suite of economic payoffs for different types of policy actions. The models consider programs that involve interactions between youth and teachers, program staff, families, and others. They show how existing and new databases can be used to analyze associations between patterns of behavior and patterns of outcomes. The sectoral costs of these outcomes can then be quantified, along with opportunities to reduce those costs through interventions with different probabilities of success. Research applying these models more comprehensively should lead to better understanding of the public and private costs and benefits of different patterns of youth risk behaviors and of investments in youth.

These analyses make it less likely that population-based actions focusing only on a single issue (e.g., smoking) will affect the young people who need the most help, compared with more comprehensive and enduring interactions. In addition to identifying the best investments in adolescent development, such analyses also can show the overall payoff to policy changes focused on the well-being of young people.

The discussants for this paper, Susan Curnan and Peter Edelman, noted its usefulness as a framework that researchers could build, expand, and adapt in revitalizing thinking about costs and benefits related to adolescent vulnerability and resiliency. Rather than focusing on adolescents as the source of troubling behaviors that drain social and institutional resources, the Burt et al. model focuses on interventions that nurture youth as assets capable of producing economic and social benefits. Curnan described a recent concrete example of such a policy, the pending bill, Younger Americans Act (H.R. 17), which aims to create *fully prepared* youth rather than *risk-free* youth. If the act were implemented, the Burt et al. model could evaluate the payoffs from potential programs. Curnan also suggested expanding the approach to include biological and community/contextual influences when profiling risk and protective factors.

Edelman pointed out that the Burt et al. model provides the ability to analyze multiple effects and interactions and could help shift intervention programs and their funding from single- to multiple-variable programs. It is thought to have potential for measuring the payoff of supporting positive youth development and improving the way we deal with adolescent vulnerability.

Adolescent Vulnerability: Measurement and Priority Setting, by Baruch Fischhoff and Henry Willis, begins by discussing adolescents' legitimate concerns about their future and well-being, reflecting their concerns about their own invulnerability. They then consider how dealing effectively with adolescent vulnerabilities requires knowing their total burden as well as the size of the component parts. The former should shape the overall investment in reducing adolescent vulnerability, the latter its allocation across interventions. Priority setting for research and practice is discussed, including the important considerations of separating facts and values when making decisions about policies and actions. The paper presents approaches to determining priorities as well as ways to determine values relevant to the particular policy choices.

Although the paper argues for setting priorities systematically, it also recognizes the challenges to this approach, such as the difficulty of the choices being faced and the political barriers to translating priorities into change in resource allocation. The proposed procedure for priority setting allows for involvement of relevant individuals, including adolescents, and not merely summaries of their views. The authors emphasize that values shape the priorities we place on young people's well-being and the procedures used to reach those priorities.

The main strength of the Fischhoff and Willis paper, according to discussants Matthew Stagner and Mark Cohen, is making transparent the assumptions, values, and uncertainties that are part of any process of risk assessment and prioritization. The paper draws attention to the multiple ways in which politics and value judgments are interwoven in the process of identifying, measuring, and creating intervention programs to address adolescent risk. In many cases, such as deciding what to measure in longitudinal studies, value judgments are the determining influence on how and where money will be spent. If choices are framed and evaluated in a scientific manner, the result should be priorities more in keeping with societal values. The Fischhoff and Willis paper offers a new way of examining how value judgments and scientific knowledge influence decision making about resources used to address adolescent vulnerability and risk. If a scientific knowledge base is available when opportunities such as public and political interest move in the direction of adolescent vulnerability, the possibility of having value judgments informed effectively by research is greater than if the research base is not present, according to Stagner. He also noted, in agreement with the other papers, the importance of developing indicators of positive development, pointing to the Federal Interagency Forum on Child and Family Statistics' *America's Children* initiative. Stagner also noted agreement with the other papers regarding creating community-specific priorities, reflecting the specificity of risks and values. The Fischhoff and Willis paper offers a way in which national and local resources might be addressed effectively to reduce adolescent vulnerability.

Mark Cohen noted the social and institutional challenges facing attempts to develop community consensus regarding which adolescent risk and evaluative factors to consider. Questions include who controls the agenda, how to select appropriate citizen participants, and how values will be combined in cases of conflict. In contrast, Cohen noted the economic approach of quantifying monetary value of those risks that can be compared across categories (Cohen, 1998). Doing so in an acceptable way could reduce the set of factors that need to be evaluated with alternative procedures capable of addressing nonmonetary concerns.

INTEGRATIVE SUMMARY

The prepared papers and ensuing discussion considered what is known, believed, and desired regarding adolescents' welfare. These realities shaped proposals for better research, communication, and action. Although entitled "adolescent vulnerability," the workshop necessarily considered the complementary and compensatory processes conferring resilience. The following themes emerged from the papers and discussions.

A Comprehensive Approach Is Needed

Looking at the full range of potential risk outcomes is essential to:

- Assess the full burden of vulnerability borne by youth and society (in terms of both direct suffering and lost potential);
- Ensure that disproportionate attention and resources are not devoted to a few of the many potentially relevant issues; and
- Identify clusters of problems with common causes and solutions.

Looking at the full range of factors creating risk and resilience is essential to:

- Assess the full impact of dislocations in young people's lives (e.g., poverty, violence);
- Assess the total contribution of interventions that might ameliorate root causes of multiple problems (e.g., creating more supportive schools, reducing social rejections, strengthening parenting skills); and
- Avoid domination by a subset of proposals.

A suite of measures of adolescents' welfare is needed to:

- Consistently track their circumstances;
- Systematically compare teens in different groups; and
- Rationally direct future resources.

Adolescents Differ in Their Needs, Wants, and Circumstances

Recognizing the differences among young people is essential to affording them the respect they deserve. Sweeping generalizations about adolescents encourage the adoption of undifferentiated interventions, with the direct costs of wasting societal resources and undermining teenagers' confidence in adults (who are ignoring significant aspects of their lives) and the opportunity costs of failing to develop better understanding and interventions.

Some adolescents face particular challenges worthy of special societal attention. These include adolescents suffering from chronic diseases, belonging to disadvantaged and disenfranchised groups (e.g., migrants, Native Americans), or dealing with psychological conditions having broad effects (e.g., depression, eating disorders).

Even within difficult situations, adolescents often find strengths in themselves and sympathetic others. Even adolescents from favored groups often experience extreme stresses (e.g., peer rejection, family disintegration). As a result, helping them may be a matter of tipping the balance in their lives, rather than creating wholesale changes in their circumstances.

Careful Research Matters

Without solid research, priorities will be set on the basis of anecdote, supposition, and prejudice. One task of research is to evaluate beliefs that are widely maintained but empirically unsupported. It cannot, however, dissuade supporters of programs that are ends in themselves (e.g., because they provide resources or a livelihood to those who administer them; because their existence expresses a social value, whatever its effects on young people).

Disentangling the interplay of risk and resilience factors requires longitudinal studies with well-selected measures and diverse samples. Properly managed and coordinated, they can provide a uniquely valuable public resource.

Effective research requires measures well matched to theoretical concepts. That applies when measuring adolescents' behavior, environmental circumstances, or beliefs, as well as beliefs about adolescents. For example, little can be concluded from many studies of risk perceptions because their questions are insufficiently precise for responses to be compared with statistical estimates of risk.

Research Must Be Communicated Effectively

Social policy and attitudes toward adolescents reflect people's beliefs about them. Often these beliefs are unfounded (e.g., adolescents have a greater sense of personal invulnerability than do adults). Such beliefs can be confronted in ways that improve public understanding of young people's vulnerability and resilience, as well as the processes shaping them.

The workings of the research community can create an unbalanced picture of adolescents, even when its results are communicated accurately. Teenagers often are studied because they face or pose problems in society. As a result, they can be unduly seen as threatened or threatening. Moreover, that research often is focused on a single problem behavior or risk factor, encouraging sweeping generalizations and simplistic solutions. Countering a fragmented view of adolescents requires either aggregating limited studies or focusing on comprehensive ones.

Many different groups and individuals are concerned with adolescents' welfare. They include parents, teachers, legislators, funders, and the young people themselves. Taking best advantage of available research requires summarizing its results, implications, and robustness in terms relevant to specific audiences. Due diligence in communication means empirically evaluating its impacts in order to ensure that it is understood as intended.

Deliberative Social Mechanisms Are Needed to Set Priorities

Sound analytical procedures are increasingly available to characterize many aspects of adolescent vulnerability. Applying these procedures more widely would provide disciplined estimates of statistics that people otherwise try to assess intuitively.

Even the most accomplished economic or risk analysis provides an imperfect estimate of a portion of the issues potentially relevant to decisions about adolescents. Moreover, the specification of such analyses inevitably requires the exercise of judgment, regarding both how to treat uncertain data and how to focus on target issues and populations. As a result, formal analyses can inform, but not determine, social choices.

Interpreting analytical results, and integrating them with other concerns, requires deliberative processes. These can create communities of concern and shared understandings (including focused disagreements) among those concerned about adolescents.

CONCLUDING THOUGHTS

As a society and as individuals, we face challenges and opportunities in providing a better future for our adolescents. The papers and discussions of this workshop have, we hope, advanced our point of departure for the work that lies ahead in setting and acting on priorities.

REFERENCES

Biehl, M., & Halpern-Felsher, B. L. (2001). Adolescents' and adults' understanding of probability expressions. *Journal of Adolescent Health 28*(1), 30-35.

Blum, R. W., Beuhring, T., Shew, M. L., Bearinger, L. H., Sieving, R. E., & Resnick, M. D. (2000). The effects of race/ethnicity, income, and family structure on adolescent risk behaviors. *American Journal of Public Health 90*(12),1879-1885.

Burt, M. R. (1998, September 16). *Reasons to invest in adolescents.* Paper prepared for the Health Futures of Youth II: Pathways to Adolescent Health, Maternal and Child Health Bureau, U.S. Department of Health and Human Services. Washington, DC: Urban Institute.

Burt, M. R., & Levy, F. (1987). Estimates of public costs for teenage childbearing: A review of recent studies and estimates of 1985 public costs. In S. L. Hofferth and C. D. Hayes (Eds.), *Risking the future: Adolescent sexuality, pregnancy, and childbearing, Vol. II, Working papers and statistical appendices* (pp. 264-293). Washington, DC: National Academy Press.

Cohen, M. A. (1998). The monetary value of saving a high-risk youth. *Journal of Quantitative Criminology, 14*(1), 5-7.

Danziger, S., & Waldfogel, J. (Eds.). (2000). *Securing the future: Investing in children from birth to college.* New York: Russell Sage Foundation.

Fischhoff, B. (1996). The real world: What good is it? *Organizational Behavior and Human Decision Processes, 65,* 232-248.

Fischhoff, B., Downs, J., & De Bruin, W. B. (1998). Adolescent vulnerability: A framework for behavioral interventions. *Applied & Preventive Psychology, 7,* 77-94.

Fischhoff, B., Parker, A. M., De Bruin, W. B., Downs, J., Palmgren, C., Daws, R., & Manski, C. (2000). Teen expectations for significant life events. *Public Opinion Quarterly, 64,* 189-205

Halpern-Felsher, B. L., Millstein, S. G., Ellen, J. M., Adler, N. E., Tschann, J. M., & Biehl, M. (2001). The role of behavioral experience in judging risks. *Health Psychology, 20,* 120-126.

Hamburg, B. A. (1982). Living with chronic illness. In T. J. Coates, A. C. Petersen, C. Perry (Eds.), *Promoting adolescent health: A dialogue on research and practice* (pp. 431-443). New York: Academic Press.

Levitt, M. Z., Selman, R. L., & Richmond, J. B. (1991). The psychosocial foundations of early adolescents' high-risk behavior: Implications for research and practice. *Journal for Research on Adolescence, 1*(4), 349-378.

Lindberg, L. D., Boggess, S., Porter, L., & Williams, S. (2000). *Teen risk taking: A statistical portrait.* Washington, DC: Urban Institute.

Masten, A. S. (2001). Ordinary magic—resilience processes in development. *American Psychologist 56,* 227-238.

Svetaz, M. V., Ireland, M., & Blum, R. (2000). Adolescents with learning disabilities: Risk and protective factors associated with emotional well being: Findings from the National Longitudinal Study of Adolescent Health. *Journal of Adolescent Health 27,* 340-348.

2

Perceptions of Risk and Vulnerability

Susan G. Millstein and Bonnie L. Halpern-Felsher

INTRODUCTION

Why Are Perceptions of Risk and Vulnerability Important?

Individuals' judgments about risk are viewed as a fundamental element of most theoretical models of health and risk behavior, including Social Cognitive Theory (Bandura, 1994), the Health Belief Model (Rosenstock, 1974), the Theory of Reasoned Action (Fishbein and Ajzen, 1975), the Theory of Planned Behavior (Ajzen, 1985), Self-Regulation Theory (Kanfer, 1970), and Subjective Culture and Interpersonal Relations Theory (Triandis, 1977). All of these theories posit that individuals' beliefs about the consequences of their actions and perceptions of their vulnerability to those consequences play a key role in behavior. Although we will later question whether existing studies address these hypotheses adequately, the strength of the logical association between risk perceptions and behavior is compelling. As a result, risk perceptions play a fundamental role in behavioral intervention programs, which try to get adolescents to recognize and acknowledge their own vulnerability to negative outcomes. The ability to judge risks also is considered to be an essential element of decision-making competence, according to theorists, researchers, and practitioners in the behavioral sciences, medicine, social work, law, and social policy (Gittler et al., 1990; Hodne, 1995).

Adults have speculated about adolescents' lack of competence in recognizing and assessing risk since the time of Aristotle. Adolescents typically are viewed as being unable to judge risk appropriately, and as having strong beliefs in their invulnerability to harm. In recent years, the question of adolescents' competence has emerged as a result of efforts to regulate the legal rights of adolescents to make decisions in the realms of medical and mental health treatment, including their rights to refuse treatment or to obtain treatment without parental knowledge and/or consent, as well as their rights to participate in research, including experimental clinical trials. Additionally, adolescents' capacity to exercise existing rights is of fundamental interest to the juvenile justice system (Butterfield, 1996).

Much of the interest in adolescents' perceptions of risk and vulnerability is motivated by the desire to understand why youth engage in potentially threatening behaviors, with an aim toward guiding the development of interventions that will be successful in preventing their onset. Relevant questions for gaining such understanding include the following:

- What skills are needed for assessing risk?
- Do adolescents have these skills?
- How competent are adolescents in identifying and assessing risk?
- What kinds of factors influence adolescents' ability to judge risk?
- How do adolescents' perceptions compare to those of adults?
- Do adolescents' perceptions of risk influence their decisions?

In this paper, we review existing data to address these questions. We acknowledge that answers to these questions will not give a complete picture of why adolescents engage in risky behavior—other crucial questions remain, such as whether adolescents are competent decision makers or able to apply their decision-making skills in all situations. Nevertheless, a focus on risk perception is a reasonable vantage point from which to consider adolescent risk and vulnerability. We will begin our discussion by giving the reader a sense of the size of the risks themselves. That is, how big are the risks that adolescents face? This will provide a context for later assessing the adequacy of adolescents' judgments concerning those risks.

How Big Are the Risks?

Some of the threats to adolescents' well-being pose sizable risks. For example, 40 percent of Latino youth fail to complete high school or the equivalent, such as the General Education Development Tests (GED) (Federal Interagency Forum on Child and Family Statistics, 2000). However, for many risks, the actual chance of a negative outcome occurring is relatively small. For example, Fischhoff et al. (2000) reported that for adolescents, the actual probability of a female getting pregnant within one year is less than 6 percent, and the probability of a male getting someone pregnant in the next year is less than 3 percent. The probability of being the victim of a violent crime (e.g., homicide, rape, robbery) is less than 10 percent. Even smaller is the probability of an adolescent dying from any cause in the next year (.08 percent) or by the time an adolescent turns 20 (.04 percent). Of course, the probability of experiencing these outcomes is highly dependent on one's behavior and environment. Risks for acquiring sexually transmitted diseases (STDs) are quite high among youth who have highly connected sexual networks involving people who live in areas of high infectivity. The risks are far lower for adolescents who live in geographic areas of low disease rates, and are essentially nil for sexually inactive youth.

But small risks are not unimportant. Although many of the actual risks adolescents face are numerically small, their potential outcomes can be severe and life altering. For example, STDs such as gonorrhea and chlamydia are associated with subsequent rates of pelvic inflammatory disease (PID) as high as 10 to 40 percent. It is estimated that of the approximately 200,000 to 400,000 adolescent females who develop PID each year, 40,000 to 84,000 of them eventually will find themselves infertile. The fiscal costs are also high; excluding costs related to HIV and AIDS, we spend an estimated $882 million yearly treating STDs in adolescents (Gans et al., 1995). Furthermore, most causes of adolescent morbidity and mortality are preventable, thus behooving us to make attempts to reduce them.

Adults' Perspectives on Adolescent Vulnerability

Although few empirical data speak directly to adults' perceptions concerning risks to adolescents, other indicators point to the sources of adults' concerns. Reading the popular press, listening to parents of teenagers, and examining the content of preventive programs makes it clear that adults' concerns focus primarily on the major causes of morbidity and mortality and adolescents' involvement in behaviors that are associated with these negative health and social outcomes. In a series of focus groups with high-risk youth, their parents and grandparents, a report from the Office of Disease Prevention and Health Promotion (1993) found that parents were concerned about the lack of adult supervision for their children and the failure of schools and communities to meet the needs of adolescents. Other areas of concern included peer influences and poor schools. Ferguson and Williams (1996) found that among a group of parents of 17 year olds, 38 percent expressed concerns about their children's driving; 43 to 97 percent of the parents supported additional restrictions to protect their children.

Parents of adolescents also view adolescents as more vulnerable than do adolescents themselves. Beyth-Marom et al. (1993) found that across a series of risky behaviors, adolescents' perceptions of the risks to themselves were significantly lower than the risks their parents perceived for them. Similar findings are reported by Cohn et al. (1995). For example, although 31 percent of the adolescents believed there was little or no harm in getting drunk once or twice, only 9 percent of the parents believed this. These formal comparisons of adults' perceptions of adolescents' risks with adolescent perceptions of their own risks is confounded by the fact that the adult is judging risks for another person—and such judgments are typically higher than personal risk judgments (Weinstein, 1980, 1983, 1984; Whalen et al., 1994).

Conceptualizing and Measuring Perceptions of Risk and Vulnerability

There are many ways to conceptualize and measure perceptions of risk and vulnerability. We can examine the content of individuals' risk and vulnerability beliefs—identifying those things that worry or concern them, as well as the degree of anxiety generated by these concerns. We can observe whether people recognize the risks inherent in a given situation, or we can look at how accurately someone judges a specific risk. Risk judgments may focus on situations (e.g., is having unprotected sex dangerous?) or on their potential outcomes (e.g., what is the chance that you will get an STD?). Personal risk can be viewed in absolute terms (e.g., what is your chance . . . ?) or relative terms (e.g., how does your risk compare to others?). For any given individual, we can also examine his or her relative ranking of the importance of various "risks" to assess his or her risk perceptions.

Each of the many ways of assessing individuals' perceptions has something to tell us about their sense of risk and vulnerability. But they also appear to measure different aspects of this construct we call vulnerability. The literature reflects this conceptual diversity, making it difficult to compare across studies. In our review, we will consider them separately. We will not attempt to tell the reader which of these approaches are best. Rather, we will comment on the use and limitations of each. To avoid confusion, we will use the following terms throughout this paper.

We use the term *risk judgment* to reflect magnitude assessments of risk. A risk judgment that focuses solely on an outcome (e.g., how likely are you to get an STD?) would be considered to be a *nonconditional risk judgment.* In contrast, a *situation-specific or conditional risk judgment* is one in which explicit mention of an antecedent condition such as a situation or a behavior is made (e.g., how likely are you to get an STD if you have unprotected sex?). When assessments of risk do not involve magnitude estimates, we use the term *risk identification.* These assessments may focus solely on a situation (e.g., is it risky to have unprotected sex?) or may include identification of specific consequences as well (e.g., what might happen if you have unprotected sex?).

Although risk identification and judgment may be the most direct ways to tap assessments of risk, individuals' affective responses to specific situations and/or outcomes also can be informative. When assessments focus on the degree of anxiety or concern individuals have about particular situations (e.g., how worried would you be if you had unprotected sex?) or outcomes (e.g., do you worry about getting an STD?), we refer to them as feelings or perceptions of *vulnerability.* Like the more cognitive aspects of risk perception, these affective manifestations can be conditional or unconditional. Asking people to identify the things that concern them (e.g., what kinds of health problems do you worry about?) points to content areas where perceptions of vulnerability may exist; we refer to these simply as *concerns.* We acknowledge that individual differences such as generalized anxiety or pessimism may influence the degree to which situations or outcomes are identified, judged, or experienced as risky. However, we do not consider these generalized states or their measurement to reflect perceptions of risk or vulnerability.

ADOLESCENTS' PERCEPTIONS

We will now review what we know about the content of adolescents' concerns, their perceptions of vulnerability, their ability to identify risk, and their ability to judge risk. In each section, we will first give the reader a sense of how adolescents as a group perform, followed by an examination of how these capacities vary by the age of the adolescent. Other sources of variation in risk perception and assessment, such as gender, race/ethnicity, and economic status, are discussed later.

Sources of Concern

One approach to understanding adolescents' perceptions of vulnerability is to identify those issues about which adolescents express concern. Numerous surveys have documented these concerns. Common adolescent concerns include those related to appearance (height, weight, acne), emotional states (depression, anxiety), interpersonal relationships (parents, friends, and other adults), school (schoolwork, school problems, and career), environmental threats (air pollution and nuclear war), and health and physical complaints (headaches, stomachaches, vision problems, dental problems). Adolescents also acknowledge the importance of the health issues most frequently identified by health professionals, including substance use, sexual behavior, birth control, sexually transmitted disease, and pregnancy (Alexander, 1989; Benedict et al., 1981; Brunswick, 1969; Giblin and Poland, 1985; Marks et al., 1983; Millstein and Irwin, 1985; Parcel et al., 1977; Sternlieb and Munan, 1972).

Although adolescents clearly acknowledge a wide range of concerns, only a few issues consistently rank high. These include issues pertaining to school, dental health, acne, interpersonal relationships, and mental health (American School Health Association et al., 1989; Sternlieb and Munan, 1972). Concerns related to substance use, sexual behavior, nutrition, and exercise rank lower in most adolescent samples (Eme et al., 1979; Feldman et al., 1986; Sobal et al., 1988).

Age Differences in Adolescents' Concerns

Observed age differences in health concerns are consistent with the developmental tasks faced by adolescents. Younger adolescents (between 11 and 13) generally are more concerned with physical development, including puberty (Byler et al., 1969), and with how one is viewed by members of the opposite sex. Middle adolescents (i.e., about 14–15 years old) are more concerned with appearance (especially among female adolescents), interpersonal relationships with peers and members of the opposite sex, and self-esteem. Older adolescents are more concerned with school, grades, and their future career plans (Eme et al., 1979; Violato and Holden, 1988) as well as their emotional health. A study of more than 5,000 children and adolescents found increasing interest among youth in topics such as growth and development, preventive health behaviors, mental health, and social-emotional development as children moved into the early adolescent years (Byler et al., 1969).

Adults' Perceptions About Adolescents' Concerns

Adults underestimate the degree of concern adolescents report about their health (Sobal et al., 1988) and appear to have misperceptions about adolescents' level of knowledge about specific topics such as AIDS (Manning and Balson, 1989). Adults also fail to recognize some of the specific health concerns of adolescents. An example occurs in regard to dental and oral health. Across studies, adolescents consistently rank dental concerns of being of great importance (Parcel et al., 1977; Sobal et al., 1988; Sternlieb and Munan, 1972). Yet this topic rarely receives attention in discussions of adolescent health. Other areas in which adults fail to recognize adolescents' concerns include school problems and teens' relationships with adults (Sobal et al., 1988).

To summarize, existing data indicate that adolescents do express concerns about negative effects that can result from volitional behaviors as well as from environmental hazards such as natural disasters, technological risks, and violence. Adults often underestimate these concerns. Although examination of adolescents' concerns gives us some indication of the sources of concern, it does not inform us about the degree to which these concerns are accompanied by feelings of vulnerability. For example, to what degree do concerns about oral health translate into adolescents' feelings of personal vulnerability to caries or gum disease? For this reason, perceptions of vulnerability may be a closer reflection of adolescents' beliefs about their vulnerability.

Perceptions of Vulnerability

Data from numerous studies indicate that adolescents feel vulnerable to experiencing negative outcomes. Adolescents' worry and feelings of vulnerability to AIDS have been well documented (DiClemente et al., 1987; Pleck et al., 1990; Price et al., 1985; Strunin, 1991). Other behavior-related risks, such as getting sick from drinking alcohol and acquiring an STD also appear to generate feelings of vulnerability. In a recent study, we found that a majority of sexually inexperienced seventh and ninth graders reported that they would be worried and concerned about getting an STD if they had sex without a condom; 53 percent said they would be very worried and 26 percent reported feeling somewhat worried. Similar percentages were obtained for adolescents' ratings of concern. Feelings of vulnerability appear to generalize beyond behavior-related risks. When asked to imagine being at a picnic when a tornado strikes, 36 percent of adolescents in seventh and ninth grade reported that they would be very worried that they would die, and 22 percent reported being somewhat worried about dying from the tornado. The corresponding values for being concerned with dying were 43 percent and 20 percent. Bachman (1983) showed that 30 percent of high school seniors reported worrying frequently about the threat of nuclear war.

Age Differences Among Adolescents

In our recent study (Millstein and Halpern-Felsher, 2001) cross-sectional analyses showed a negative relationship between age and feelings of vulnerability to alcohol (r=–.30) and sex risks (–.35). Feelings of vulnerability to alcohol-caused illness were significantly higher in fifth and seventh graders than ninth graders and adults. Perceptions of vulnerability to STDs were significantly higher in seventh and ninth graders than adults. Longitudinal analyses (in progress) showed that among sexually inexperienced seventh and ninth graders, worry over getting an STD as a result of unprotected sex decreased significantly over a 6-month period. However, reported concern for STDs did not. Additional data supporting these findings are provided by data from the National Survey of Adolescent Males (Pleck et al., 1993), which showed that adolescent males' (ages 15–19) worry about AIDS decreased over a two-year period.

Thus, in contrast to popular views that adolescents do not worry or concern themselves about risks, the data indicate that many, and in some cases most, adolescents report feeling vulnerable to negative outcomes. It is not entirely clear, however, what these assessments really mean. Do they reflect true anxiety and/or perceptions of potential harm, or are they primarily cognitive expressions, meant to acknowledge that these are things, in general, to worry about? Who, after all, does not worry (at least academically) about negative outcomes such as AIDS?

Risk Identification

Studies of adolescents' capacity for considering consequences have shown that even young adolescents have the ability to identify negative consequences associated with medical procedures (Kaser-Boyd et al., 1985; Lewis, 1981; Weithorn and Campbell, 1982) and with engaging in risky behaviors (Beyth-Marom et al., 1993; Finn and Brown, 1981; Furby et al., 1997). Typically, these studies ask participants to imagine themselves in a hypothetical situation, and to identify any risks that they perceive in that situation. For example, Beyth-Marom et al. (1993) asked adolescents to consider what might happen if they engaged in six different risky activities. They found that adolescents identified, on average, four to seven consequences for each activity. A broad range of consequences were mentioned, including physical effects, psychological effects, and social reactions from family, other authority figures, and peers.

A few studies have examined the extent to which adolescents spontaneously mention or consider risks, which may give a more realistic picture of adolescents' ability to recognize risk in real-life situations. Lewis (1981) asked 108 adolescents in grades 7, 8, 10, and 12 about the advice they would give to peers facing cosmetic surgery and to peers considering participation in a clinical trial of a new acne medicine. Sixty percent of the adolescents mentioned possible risks associated with the situations, and 26 percent mentioned potential future consequences. Halpern-Felsher and Cauffman (2001) used the same scenarios in their study of 190 adolescents (grades 6, 8, 10, and 12). They found that 12 to 32 percent of teens mentioned risks and 10 to 13 percent mentioned future consequences in the cosmetic surgery scenario. In the informed consent scenario, 42 to 63 percent of the adolescents recognized risks and 7 to 16 percent recognized future consequences.

Age Differences in Risk Identification

Studies examining age differences in adolescents' ability to identify risks report conflicting findings. Lewis (1981) found dramatic increases in awareness of risks between grades 10 (50 percent of subjects mentioning) and 12 (83 percent). Mention of future consequences showed steady increases over grades 7–8 (11 percent), 10 (25 percent), and 12 (42 percent). However, a replication of the Lewis study using a somewhat larger sample (Halpern-Felsher and Cauffman, 2001) reported no significant age differences in adolescents' consideration of risks and long-term consequences. Two other studies also failed to find age differences. In a small sample (N=62) of people with learning and behavior problems, Kaser-Boyd et al. (1985) found younger adolescents to be as competent as older adolescents in their ability to consider consequences. Ambuel (1992) studied 13 to 21 year olds (N=75) who suspected an unplanned pregnancy and were seeking a pregnancy test. Comparisons between younger minors (ages 13–15 years) and older minors (16-17) showed no differences in their consideration of consequences.

In four studies focusing on risk identification that compared adolescents and adults, two found adults to be more competent in identifying risk. Beyth-Marom et al. (1993) reported small age-related differences in subjects' ability to generate consequences associated with six risky behaviors, with adults spontaneously mentioning more consequences than adolescents on one-third of the behaviors examined. Halpern-Felsher and Cauffman (2001) found that in comparison to adolescents, adults considered a greater number of risks as well as long-term consequences. Both of these studies used hypothetical situations to estimate participants' capacity for identifying risk. In contrast, the other two studies focusing on risk identification examined perceptions of risk in real life decision-making situations and failed to find differences between adolescents and adults in their ability to consider consequences (Ambuel, 1992; Kaser-Boyd et al., 1985). Both samples were relatively small, including fewer than 80 participants.

To summarize, it is clear that many adolescents, especially older adolescents, are capable of recognizing and identifying risks. Adolescents also are able to identify risks spontaneously, in response to hypothetical scenarios as well as in real-life decision situations. However, the overall level of competence among adolescents is not exceptionally high. In the Lewis (1981) study, few of the younger adolescents and less than half of the tenth graders could be considered competent in identifying important potential risks. Halpern-Felsher and Cauffman (2001) also reported lower than expected levels of awareness of risks among both adolescents and adults. Furthermore, most studies that have examined age differences in risk identification report age-related increases in individuals' awareness and consideration of risks (Ambuel, 1992; Beyth-Marom et al., 1993; Lewis, 1981); fewer have failed to find such differences (Lewis, 1980; Weithorn and Campbell, 1982). Although it is not clear whether there are absolute points at which one should be considered competent in identifying risks, the finding of age-related increases in risk identification does call into question the degree to which we should consider adolescents, particularly younger adolescents, competent. The extent to which the ability to identify risks changes over time has not been studied using longitudinal data, nor has the link between risk identification and risk behavior been studied.

Risk Judgments

In addressing whether adolescents are able to judge risks accurately, one can use a number of different indicators. One indicator might be to look at whether adolescents view themselves as "invulnerable," a common attribution that would render them unable to judge risks adequately. If we interpret invulnerability as meaning that the individual judges risk as nonexistent (i.e., risk estimates of zero-percent chance), research does not support this characterization of adolescents. Both Quadrel et al. (1993) and Millstein and Halpern-Felsher (2001) found perceptions of invulnerability to characterize a minority of the adolescents they sampled.

Ideally, we would judge adolescents' competence in assessing risk by comparing their perceptions to their actual risk status. But determining an individual's risk for experiencing a specific negative outcome is difficult because it depends on so many individual and environmental factors. Two people drinking the same amount of alcohol and getting into their car to drive can have very different probabilities of having an accident, depending on their body weight, food consumption, level of tolerance for alcohol, weather conditions, and so on. Similarly, the risk of pregnancy depends on factors, such as the individual's age, history of sexually transmitted disease, stage in the menstrual cycle, and type and extent of contraceptive use.

Because of the complexity in ascertaining risk status, estimates of individuals' risks often are based on aggregated risk. Thus, for example, we might judge an adolescent's risk of acquiring an STD as a function of the incidence of STDs in sexually active adolescents. Using this approach, Fischhoff et al. (2000) compared adolescents' risk judgments with data for estimating actual risk. Their sample included more than 3,500 15 to 16 year old adolescents from the 1997 National Longitudinal Study of Youth. The adolescents were asked to judge the probability that they would experience specific outcomes (i.e., risk judgments were nonconditional). The comparisons indicated that, as a group, adolescents' estimates were fairly accurate for some events (such as being in school one year later or becoming pregnant over the next year). For example, adolescents estimated their chance of experiencing or causing pregnancy within the year as 6.3 percent, which is very close to the actual probability of less than 6 percent. They were slightly optimistic about their chances of obtaining a high school diploma and getting a 4-year college degree. They were pessimistic about their estimates concerning the probability of serving time in jail or prison, judging the likelihood at 5 percent, which is nearly 10 times higher than the actual probability of 0.6 percent. They greatly overestimated their chances of dying in the next year or by their twentieth birthday, judging the probability as 18.6 percent, while in actuality it is less than 1 percent. Of course, as averages, these estimates do not inform us about the proportion of adolescents who are accurate. Examination of the distribution of percentage estimates indicates that although adolescents as a group appeared to have reasonable estimates in many areas, few individuals in the sample actually demonstrated an accurate sense of risk.

Even in the absence of comparisons such as these, there are indications that adolescents are quite inaccurate in estimating risk. When we examine adolescents' quantitative estimates and compare them with even approximate probability estimates, we find that adolescents overestimate risk. For example, Halpern-Felsher et al. (2001) reported that nonsexually active adolescents and young adults estimated their chance of getting an STD if they had unprotected sex once as 44 percent, and the chance of contracting HIV/AIDS given the same situation as 38 percent. Participants who had never used alcohol estimated a 79-percent chance of getting into an accident if they drove with a drunk driver. It is possible that adolescents' high risk judgments can be explained by their inability to understand and use quantitative percentages. However, analyses controlling for adolescents' skill in understanding percentages continue to yield high estimates (Millstein and Halpern-Felsher, 2001).

Methods for estimating adolescents' competence also have included the use of comparative risk assessments. These assessments ask people to estimate whether their chance of experiencing an outcome is higher, the same, or lower than other people like themselves. The rationale is that, in a given population, some people's risk will be higher than others, some will be lower than others, and some will be the same as others. Not everyone can be at lower risk. Given this, the mean comparative risk assessment at the aggregate level should be normally distributed. However, studies generally find that, as a group, adolescents (as well as adults) bias their assessments in the direction of viewing their risk as lower than the risk for similar others (Whalen et al., 1994).

Age Differences in Risk Judgments

Earlier, we noted that risk judgments could be nonconditional or conditional. When we move to review age differences in judgments of personal risk, the distinction between these types of risk assessments becomes particularly important. To illustrate the fundamental difference between these kinds of assessments, let us consider risk judgments concerning lung cancer. A nonconditional risk judgment asks the individual to judge his or her risk of developing lung cancer, without specifying any potential situational factors that might be relevant. If we ask a nonsmoker to judge his or her risk of developing lung cancer, the response would reflect his or her assessment of the likelihood that a nonsmoker will develop lung cancer. But if we ask the same question of a smoker, his or her assessment would reflect a judgment about the likelihood that a smoker will develop lung cancer. Nonconditional assessments thus pose a problem of interpretation because they assess different things as a function of the respondent's behavioral experience.

An alternative method for eliciting risk judgments is to have individuals judge their risk under specific situations or conditions. Asking individuals to judge their risk of developing lung cancer *if they smoked cigarettes* represents what we call a conditional risk judgment (see Halpern-Felsher et al., 2001). Regardless of one's own smoking status, individuals are responding to the same question and are asked to make the same assessment. These risk judgments are more useful as their meaning is less dependent on factors such as the behavioral characteristics of the respondent (Ronis, 1992; Van der Velde et al., 1996).

The use of nonconditional risk judgments is especially troubling in studies examining age differences in risk perception because experience is a known source of variation in risk judgment (Gerrard et al., 1996b; Van der Plight, 1998) that varies by age as well. For this reason, we will limit our review and commentary to studies that either elicit conditional risk judgments or control for behavioral experience if using nonconditional risk judgments. Thus, we will not comment on some frequently cited studies such as those reported by Gochman and Saucier (1982).

Three investigations have studied age differences in adolescents using conditional assessments of risk. Of them, only Cohn et al. (1995) failed to find age differences among adolescents. Urberg and Robbins (1984) found that perceptions of smoking-related risks had a curvilinear relationship to age in a sample of adolescents in grades 6 through 12. A strong inverse relationship was characteristic of adolescents in grades 6 through 8; and a smaller, positive relationship was found among adolescents in grades 8 through 12. Results from our recent work (Millstein and Halpern-Felsher, 2001), which examined risk judgments across a range of domains, suggest a more linear, negative relationship with age, with older adolescents' judgments of risk significantly lower than those of younger adolescents.

Although these cross-sectional studies suggest the possibility of age differences in risk judgment, only longitudinal studies that examine changes within subjects over time can tell us whether these differences are truly developmentally based or due to cohort differences. Only our study offers such longitudinal data using conditional risk judgments. Analyses are still in progress. However, preliminary analyses of adolescents' risk judgment for STDs indicate that among sexually inexperienced ninth graders, there is a significant decrease over a one-year period in their perceived risk of personally getting an STD if they have unprotected sex (from a mean risk judgment of 43 percent to a mean of 36 percent). We saw no significant changes in the seventh graders' risk judgments over the one-year period.

A number of differences among these studies are worth noting. Although all of the studies specified particular situational conditions, their specificity differed. Urberg and Robbins (1984) queried subjects about risks "if you smoked regularly." Cohn et al. (1995) asked about risks associated with engaging in a behavior once or twice. We used highly detailed scenarios to minimize variability in how participants would interpret underspecified risk situations (Fischhoff, 1996) and to assure that risk judgment differences were not a function of such interpretive differences (Biehl and Halpern-Felsher, 2001; Ellen et al., 1998; Fischoff, 1996). For example, in the scenario designed to elicit judgments about risks for STD, the risk situation (having unprotected sex) specified both the type of sexual partner as well as the number of unprotected episodes of sex.

Comparisons of Adolescents and Adults

A reasonable indicator for judging adolescents' competence in assessing risks is to compare their performance with that of adults because adults generally are considered competent in the eyes of the law. It can also shed light on potential developmental differences in the ability to judge risks. A small number of studies provide such adolescent-adult comparisons. Cohn et al. (1995) found adolescents to rate their risk of harm as lower than did their parents. But two other studies support the idea that adolescents perceive greater risk than adults. Quadrel et al. (1993) had adolescents and their parents assess the probability of experiencing a variety of behavior-linked negative outcomes. Defining absolute invulnerability as the belief that one faces no risk (i.e., zero-percent probability) of experiencing particular outcomes, they found that adolescents were less likely to judge themselves as invulnerable than were their parents. Similarly, Millstein and Halpern-Felsher (2001) found that a significantly greater proportion of adults demonstrated perceptions of absolute invulnerability (34 percent) than did adolescents (14 percent). Additionally, we found that adolescents' risk judgments were significantly higher than those of adults' judgments across a range of natural hazards and behavior-linked outcomes. The magnitude and direction of the findings remained consistent across different types of risk judgment measures. The differences also remained significant after controlling for experience with the behavior and the negative outcomes.

A number of additional studies provide information about differences in risk perceptions between adolescents and adults. Perceptions of risks to other children (not personal risk assessments) were examined by McClure-Martinez and Cohn (1996), who found perceptions of risk of childhood injury to be higher among adolescent mothers than older mothers. Sastre et al. (1999) found adolescents (ages 15–20) to be more accurate than adults in perceiving a linear dose-risk relationship for smoking cigarettes. Goldberg et al. (2001a) found adolescents to make more heuristically based errors than adults in their judgments of risk. Quadrel et al. (1993) had adolescents and their parents assess the probability of experiencing a variety of behavior-linked negative outcomes. They found that adolescents were less likely to judge themselves as absolutely invulnerable than were their parents. Similarly, Millstein and Halpern-Felsher (2001) found that a significantly greater proportion of adults demonstrated perceptions of absolute invulnerability (34 percent) than did adolescents (14 percent).

Overall then, research to date shows that many, and in some cases most, adolescents report feeling some degree of vulnerability to negative outcomes and few evidence perceptions that they are invulnerable to harm. In fact, most studies show perceptions of decreased risk with age (Bernstein and Woodall, 1987; Millstein and Halpern-Felsher, 2001; Quadrel et al., 1993); judgments of risk are greatest in younger adolescents, and greater in adolescents than in adults. Although we do not yet have longitudinal data to inform us about whether these differences represent actual developmental phenomena, we believe they may well be, given what we know about other aspects of development. In the section of this paper entitled "Risk Judgment: A Developmental-Ecological Perspective," we discuss how cognitive and psychosocial development, coupled with social experiences, could suggest that this is the case. However, in interpreting these findings, it is essential to consider what judgments of risk actually represent. If we construe them to represent perceptions of vulnerability, research points to a heightened sense of vulnerability in adolescents compared to adults. If we view risk judgments as literal expressions of risk status, a different picture emerges—one of adolescents as far less accurate than adults.

Demographic Correlates of Risk and Vulnerability Perceptions

Several individual-level demographic factors have been hypothesized to influence perceptions of risk and vulnerability, including gender, race/ethnicity, and socioeconomic status. With the exception of gender, few studies have been conducted; these are reviewed in the following paragraphs.

Gender Differences

There are fairly consistent gender differences in adolescents' health concerns, perceptions of vulnerability, and perceptions of risk. Across studies representing a diversity of samples, females consistently report thinking more about their health and having more health concerns than do males (Alexander, 1989; Brunswick and Josephson, 1972; Feldman et al., 1986; Parcel et al., 1977; Porteous, 1979; Radius et al., 1980; Sobal et al., 1988; University of Minnesota, 1989; Violato and Holden, 1988).

Females also judge risks as being more likely than do males. Adolescent females (17–20) perceived greater risks and fewer benefits associated with drug use, alcohol use, and sexual behavior than did adolescent males (Parsons et al., 1997). Across a number of well-specified driving situations, including situations involving the use of alcohol, Mundt et al. (1992) found that older adolescent females (18–20) rated the probability of getting into a serious driving accident as more likely than did the males. These differences appear to persist into adulthood. In a study of parents of 17 year olds, mothers were more concerned about driving-related safety issues for their children than were fathers (Ferguson and Williams, 1996).

Gender differences also emerge in cross-cultural studies. Kassinove and Sukhodolsky (1995) compared American and Russian adolescents (ages 10 to 18) concerning the degree to which they worry about 13 outcomes, such as developing cancer, being a victim of a violent crime, poor grades, and dying, as well 6 items concerning global worry, such as world hunger, overpopulation of the planet, and environmental pollution. In both the Russian and American samples, adolescent females worried more about both personal and global issues than did their male counterparts. Similar gender differences have been found in Swedish studies (Drottz-Sjoberg and Sjoberg, 1991).

Racial/Ethnic Differences

Few studies have examined differences in health concerns and perceptions of risk as a function of race or ethnicity, and even fewer have disentangled the effects of social class or economic status in their analyses. The limited research available generally shows that in comparison with white adolescents, black adolescents think more about their health (American Cancer Society, 1979; Sobal et al., 1988), have more health concerns (Sobal et al., 1988), are more concerned about future illness (American Cancer Society, 1979), and believe they are more susceptible to specific health outcomes, such as cancer (Price et al., 1988). There are some exceptions, however. Ey et al. (2000) found that Caucasian adolescents (11–19 year olds) perceived themselves at more risk for stroke, cancer, heart attack, and motor vehicle accident than did their African American counterparts.

Differences also emerge in the nature of the specific concerns. Black adolescents have been found to be more concerned about substance use than white adolescents (Alexander, 1989). Concerns about mental health may show a different pattern, with white adolescents reporting mental health concerns more often than Hispanic or black adolescents (Parcel et al., 1977).

Actual differences in health status among white, black, and Hispanic youth could explain some of these perceptions, particularly about threats to health. But this is unlikely to explain all of the differences. For example, Strunin (1991) found Asian adolescents to be more worried about getting AIDS than were Caucasian adolescents, despite their far lower rates of sexual activity and infection. Futhermore, because health status is tied so closely to economic status and minorities are generally less economically advantaged, it is not clear whether these racial/ethnic differences would persist or new ones would emerge in studies controlling for economic status.

Economic Differences

Surprisingly little is known about how economic conditions influence adolescents' perceptions about the world (see Bloom-Feshbach et al., 1982, for a review). Two studies reported no differences in perceptions of risk and vulnerability to health problems as a function of socioeconomic status (Gochman and Saucier, 1982; Michielutte and Diseker, 1982). Yet we would expect the broad environmental context of adolescents' lives to influence their general perceptions of the world, including their perceptions of risk. In their comparison of American and Russian adolescents, Kassinove and Sukhodolsky (1995) found that the Russian adolescents were significantly more worried than the American students on both the personal and global worry scales. Similarly, the concerns that predominate in adolescents' lives have been shown to vary over generations as a function of social and economic factors that members of different cohorts experience (Natapoff and Essoka, 1989; Porteous, 1979).

THE RELATIONSHIP OF BELIEFS AND BEHAVIOR

Do Perceptions of Risk and Vulnerability Influence Behavior?

Perceptions of risk are viewed as playing a central role in motivating adolescents' behavior. To validate this hypothesis, one would want to study people *before* they began to engage in risk behavior. We would examine their beliefs about the risks they would face if they engaged in the behavior (i.e., conditional risk assessments), and then would follow them longitudinally to see whether they eventually engage in the specific behavior. Theoretically, those people who perceived less risk and/or felt less vulnerable to negative outcomes would be more likely to end up engaging in the behavior than those who initially perceived higher risk.

Given the broad implications of a causal link between risk judgment and risky behavior, one is struck by the absence of such studies in the literature. Instead, a typical research paradigm has been to look at differences in risk judgment between people who engage in risky behavior ("engagers") and those who do not ("nonengagers"). For example, studies have examined differences between smokers' and nonsmokers' judgments of risk for getting lung cancer or have compared personal risk estimates of contracting HIV among individuals who do and do not engage in unsafe sex. These studies found that individuals with behavioral experience rate their risk of experiencing negative outcomes as *higher* than do nonengagers (Cohn et al., 1995; Gerrard et al., 1996b; Gladis et al., 1992; McKenna et al., 1993; Moore and Rosenthal, 1991, 1992). Given the use of nonconditional assessments (e.g., "What is your risk of developing lung cancer?")

and a cross-sectional design, it is no surprise to find that smokers perceived themselves as being at higher risk for developing lung cancer than do non-smokers. But when we ask people about their personal risk, were they to engage in a specific behavior (e.g., "What is your risk of developing lung cancer if you smoke?"), we find *lower* judgments of risk among people who are engaging in risky behaviors (Benthin et al., 1993; Halpern-Felsher et al., 2001; Urberg and Robbins, 1984). In other words, engagers perceive the risks of engaging in the behavior as lower.

Together, this set of studies suggests that people who are engaging in risky behavior recognize that these behaviors entail risk, but view the risks as less significant than do people who do not engage in the risks. The cross-sectional nature of these studies means, of course, that we do not know whether those who engage in risky behavior perceived lower risk *prior to the onset* of the behaviors. Thus, they cannot answer the question of whether risk judgments influenced the behavior, as is hypothesized by models of health behavior, or whether the risk judgments being assessed in these studies reflect behavioral experiences—a plausible alternative hypothesis that we will entertain later (Finn and Brown, 1981; Gerrard et al., 1996a, 1996b; Halpern-Felsher et al., 2001; Urberg and Robbins, 1984). Of course, if the relationship between perceptions of risk and involvement in risky behavior is a reciprocal one (which we believe is the case), both hypotheses could be true, with judgments of risk influencing behavior as well as experience playing a role in how people view risk. Showing these kinds of effects would require fairly lengthy longitudinal studies, as one would have to recruit people prior to the onset of risky behaviors, and follow them long enough for negative outcomes[1] to have occurred to them or at least experienced vicariously. Ideally, these studies would begin early enough to investigate the role that cognitive development plays (i.e., in very early adolescence, around the age of 10) and be followed into early adulthood, with frequent assessments of adolescents' behaviors, experiences with negative outcomes, and risk judgments. If such studies were con-

[1]Experiencing negative outcomes, either vicariously (Weinstein, 1989) or personally (Roe-Berning and Straker, 1997), is associated with perceptions of higher personal risk. For many risky behaviors, few adolescents will experience negative outcomes, thus making it difficult to ascertain the effects of negative outcomes on behavior. However, outcomes such as sexually transmitted diseases are prevalent enough to make their study possible, at least in terms of understanding the role of direct personal experience.

ducted, we would expect to find a reciprocal relationship between risk judgments and experience.

It is important to recognize that risk perceptions are but one of many factors influencing behavior. Intervention programs invest a great deal of energy attempting to influence adolescents' perceptions of risk. The assumption is that given the knowledge that specific behaviors entail risk, adolescents will avoid those behaviors. Yet the relatively high overestimates of risk we see in adolescents should alert us to the suspicion that this explanation may be an overly simplistic one. A more reasonable way to view perceptions of risk is that they are necessary for motivating protective behavior, but they are not sufficient. It is unlikely that someone purposely will avoid a potentially pleasurable activity if he or she perceives absolutely no risk in doing so. But simply perceiving risk may not be sufficient. Indeed, although behavioral and decision-making models propose a key role for risk perception, they also articulate other critical influences on behavior, such as perceptions of benefits.

The Role of Perceived Benefits

The theoretical importance of benefits is recognized in the decision-making literature, which posits that individuals consider both risks and benefits (e.g., a cost-benefit model) when making decisions (compare to Baron, 1988; Weinstein and Fineberg, 1980). Benefits also are highlighted in theories of health-related behaviors, and have been shown to be an important predictor of drinking behavior (Christiansen et al., 1989; Smith et al., 1995).

Goldberg et al. (2001b) found that with increasing age and experience, adolescent respondents perceived the benefits of alcohol to be more likely and the risks to be less likely. The perceived benefits of alcohol became a more important predictor than risks in adolescents' intentions to drink alcohol across age groups and levels of experience. Among respondents who drank, the vast majority reported experiencing consequences that were positive. Furthermore, as an indication of the robust nature of this finding, this pattern of results was replicated with respondents' self-generated responses about alcohol and in the context of another health-threatening behavior, cigarette smoking. These results are in contrast to the messages adolescents typically receive about risk behavior, which are mainly about the negative, and often fatal, results. The authors argue that the failure to experience even minor negative outcomes, combined with the unexpected experience of positive outcomes, may have caused the benefits to loom larger in adolescents' decision making.

Goldberg et al. (2001b) also argue that rather than interpreting the relatively smaller risk estimates of older respondents as biased perceptions of "invulnerability," a better explanation is that they are adjusting their perceptions on the basis of both their positive experiences and the failure to experience negative outcomes. They present data to support this "adjustment" interpretation. Examining open-ended responses concerning the bad and good things that could happen from drinking alcohol, they found that from fifth graders through the adults, there were progressively fewer respondents who said there was "nothing" good about drinking alcohol (28 percent of fifth graders, 16 percent of seventh graders, 9 percent of ninth graders, and 2 percent of adults). If one includes the "missing" responses, which may well indicate that the respondents did not think there was any good that could result from drinking, the adjustment is even more dramatic: 38 percent of fifth graders, 24 percent of seventh graders, 12 percent of ninth graders, and 3 percent of adults.

Other studies have found similar results. Urberg and Robbins (1981) found significant differences in both perceived costs and perceived benefits between 12 to 15 year old nonsmokers who intended to smoke and those with no smoking intentions; adolescents with intentions to smoke perceived more benefits and fewer costs than their counterparts. Covington and Omelich (1992) examined perceived risks and benefits to smoking between regular smokers and nonsmoking sixth, eighth, and tenth graders and also found that regular smokers perceived fewer costs and more benefits than did nonsmokers. Furthermore, they reported that the perception of risks decreased with age.

We can see from this discussion concerning benefits that it is important to understand the kinds of outcomes valued by adolescents. Health concerns may not rank as high as social concerns. Understanding the interplay between perceived risks and benefits highlights the importance of recognizing that people value different things. All other things being equal, individuals are more likely to take risks if they stand to gain highly valued outcomes (benefits). Similarly, they are more likely to avoid risks when they stand to lose highly valued outcomes. There are, of course, individual differences in determining what it is that people value.

Summary of the Relationship Between Beliefs and Behavior

Studies assessing whether risk judgments are sensitive to behavioral experiences have yielded different results depending on the type of risk assessment measure used. The majority of studies have used nonconditional measures and find that individuals' estimates concerning the likelihood that they will experience a particular negative outcome (e.g., STDs) is higher among those who engage in risky behaviors linked to the outcome (i.e., unprotected sex) than among those who do not engage in the risky behavior. The few studies that have used conditional risk assessments find that adolescents who have engaged in a risk behavior perceive less risk than do nonengagers. The degree to which these associations are causal or the direction of the associations cannot be determined due to the cross-sectional designs used.

Furthermore, few studies have empirically examined other factors that might be playing a role in adolescents' decisions to engage in risk behavior, such as perceived benefits or the value, importance, or severity of different negative and positive outcomes.

RISK JUDGMENT: A DEVELOPMENTAL-ECOLOGICAL PERSPECTIVE

We have described how judgments of risk can vary among individuals, as well as how behavioral experiences and the social environment can influence these perceptions. But the information we have presented is static; it does not integrate what we know about the enormous changes that take place during the adolescent years as a function of cognitive development, psychosocial development, and changes in the nature of the social environment. Only by bringing in a developmental-ecological perspective can we integrate what is currently known to help us understand how risk perception may change over time, the effects of experience at different periods, and the role that behavioral experiences may play.

Judging risks involves an assessment of the degree to which a given antecedent is causally linked to a particular consequence or outcome. Understanding and assessing correlational evidence and making judgments about causal relationships requires the ability to process a large array of data (e.g., processing information about all possible combinations of antecedents and outcomes), as well as metacognitive skills needed to integrate new information relevant to one's own theories about causal relationships. Young adolescents have a limited ability to coordinate information, attend to smaller portions of available data (Byrnes et al., 1999; Inhelder and Piaget, 1958; Shaklee and Goldston, 1989), and tend to think in fewer dimensions than older adolescents (Piaget, 1971). Additionally, although younger adolescents are able to use theories about causal relationships, they generally are not equipped to reflect on those theories. As a result, younger adolescents are less able to consider the possibility that a contingency is false, or to consider that alternative causal relations are possible (Kuhn et al., 1988). This would suggest that younger adolescents would be more likely than older adolescents or adults to believe what they have been taught about causal relationships between risky behaviors and negative outcomes—namely, that engaging in these behaviors entails significant risk.

As adolescents mature, they become better able to entertain the possibility that a particular contingency is false. Through observation, they also learn about the relationship of risk behaviors and negative outcomes. Even if an adolescent has not engaged in risk behavior, the exposure to risky behavior increases dramatically over time as a result of the number of peers who engage in these behaviors (Centers for Disease Control and Prevention, 1998). Because most experiences with risk behaviors do not lead to negative outcomes, few examples of these outcomes are likely to have been observed. Adolescents who have just begun to think about theories of causality have great difficulty integrating such information and recognizing that there can be exceptions to the rule (Kuhn et al., 1988). Psychosocial development may also provide adolescents with further impetus for questioning what they have been taught. They have greater needs for autonomy, which often translate into their desires for autonomous decision making (Connell and Halpern-Felsher, 1997; Midgley and Feldlaufer, 1987; Steinberg and Silverberg, 1986). Challenging adults' teachings about the risks of particular behaviors could be one way in which such needs are expressed.

The development of thinking skills and changes in how information is processed appears to continue throughout the adolescent years and into young adulthood. However, not all of these developmental changes point to increased rationality. Jacobs and Potenza (1991), Davidson (1995), and Reyna and Ellis (1994) show that classical decision-making biases, such as the use of the representativeness heuristic, increase between childhood and adulthood. The ways in which people deal with evidence of noncovariation appears to improve with subsequent development (Kuhn et al., 1988), but remains suboptimal and shows increasing evidence of motivational bias.

People process outcomes and evidence in ways that reflect their underlying theories (Klaczynski and Narasimham, 1998; Kuhn, 1992). In particular, they uncritically accept evidence in favor of their views while spending a considerable amount of time finding flaws in evidence that is contrary to their views. This suggests that even when people confront evidence that risk behaviors can lead to negative outcomes (e.g., through increases in their vicarious exposure to negative outcomes), they would maintain their theories of low perceived risk rather than to react with judgments of increased risk.

In the absence of personal experience with risk behaviors, cognitive and psychosocial development, along with changes in the social environment, could thus explain why younger adolescents perceive risks as being so high, and why judgments of risk appear lower among older adolescents and young adults. If the age group differences we see are indeed developmental in nature, it would suggest a natural tendency for risk judgments to decrease over time.

Against such a backdrop, now let us imagine what might happen if an adolescent began to engage in risky behavior. The probability that he or she actually would experience a negative outcome is relatively low. Additionally, the probability of experiencing positive effects and benefits would be relatively high. In the absence of experiencing negative outcomes, we would expect to see adolescents' perceptions of risk show even more dramatic decreases. Preliminary data from our longitudinal study hint at such an effect. Among adolescents who were not sexually active, we saw significant decreases over a one-year period in their perceptions of personal risk for STDs and HIV (decreases of 8 percent and 9 percent, respectively). However, the corresponding decreases among adolescents who became sexually active during the same time period were even greater (15 percent and 21 percent, respectively). Therefore, although both groups demonstrated a decrease in risk judgments over the one-year period, the amount of change was significantly larger among adolescents who began to engage in a risky behavior and did not experience a negative outcome.

It is possible the lower judgments of risk in adults get their impetus from age-related increases in susceptibility to inferential biases. Investigators who have found increases in decision-making biases between childhood and adulthood suggest that this increase is due to their acquisition of certain knowledge structures. For example, Davidson (1995) shows that young people are more likely to show the representativeness bias (as it applies to scenarios about the elderly) after they become aware of stereotypes about the elderly. Decreasing judgments of risk also may reflect greater awareness of actual probabilities (which are generally low) and a move toward greater accuracy in older individuals. These are questions to be explored in further research.

CONCLUSIONS AND NEXT STEPS

Ultimately, we are interested in understanding why adolescents make the decisions they do and their competence in making these decisions. Why do adolescents engage in potentially threatening behaviors? Are they able to make informed decisions about undergoing or foregoing potentially dangerous medical treatments? Should we be granting them more legal rights or should they be more restricted? In considering adolescents' perceptions of risk and vulnerability, we are acknowledging the importance of these perceptions in addressing these larger questions. Existing research has offered us insights into how adolescents view risk and vulnerability, identified some of the important correlates of these constructs, and raised interesting questions concerning the effects of these perceptions on adolescents' behavior. It also has suggested to us some important next steps for a comprehensive research agenda and for program development, and some implications for a broad range of social policies concerning adolescents.

Despite strong beliefs to the contrary, there is little in the scientific literature to indicate that adolescents see themselves as invulnerable to harm. If anything, they appear to overestimate many of the risks around them. Given this, we believe that efforts to decrease public and scientific perceptions of "the invulnerable adolescent" may be warranted. As noted by others (Beyth-Marom et al., 1993; Hamburg et al., 1993), we may be doing adolescents a disservice by perpetuating this myth. Perceptions of "the invulnerable adolescent" could, for example, have negative influences on policy or funding priorities relating to adolescents. It becomes much easier for policy makers to believe that adolescent interventions are futile if they have been convinced that adolescents are destined to see themselves as invulnerable.

Although we see little evidence to suggest that adolescents perceive themselves as invulnerable to harm, existing data are more ambiguous when it comes to the question of adolescents' actual competence in identifying and judging risk. Most studies report age-related increases in individuals' awareness and consideration of risks, with adults showing greater awareness than adolescents. Depending on the standards used, adolescents' competence in identifying risk does not appear to be exceptionally high. Furthermore, if we consider risk judgments to be measures of accuracy, age is associated with greater accuracy, and adults are more accurate (and thus more competent) than adolescents. Given that adults are generally more knowledgeable than adolescents, such an interpretation is reasonable.

On the other hand, if we choose to interpret risk judgments as reflections of individuals' sense of vulnerability, it would suggest that the young feel more vulnerable than older adolescents, and adolescents feel more vulnerable than adults. Given the consistency of age differences across different types of risk, it seems plausible to suggest the possibility that individuals' risk judgments do reflect generalized feelings of vulnerability or anxiety, and that such feelings are greater among the young. Such an interpretation is reasonable in light of changes in cognitive development and exposure to a changing social environment and also suggests to us that more attention be paid to the more affective dimensions of risk perception.

Caution is warranted in interpreting these results, however, because of serious concerns about whether the research paradigms used to study risk perception are able to give us an adequate picture of how adolescents judge risks in real situations. Most studies utilize hypothetical scenarios, which carry little of the emotion-arousing potential of real situations. Real-world studies have the advantage of offering contextually accurate settings but are often of limited generalizability due to their use of highly selected samples. Laboratory-based studies offer control and the ability to look for generalizable processes, but lack ecological validity. As a result, there has been a call for efforts to create more realistic, "real-world" simulations that would offer the advantages of laboratory research while maintaining salience and ecological validity (e.g., Ebbesen and Konecni, 1980). Such studies also could provide a means of more accurately measuring the affective components of risk perception.

The need for definitive studies concerning the risk perception-risk behavior relationship cannot be overstated. Because of the theoretical importance of the perceived risk construct to behavior, prevention and intervention programs frequently invest a great deal of effort trying to get adolescents to recognize and acknowledge their own vulnerability to negative outcomes. Such approaches are supported by experimental studies that have shown it is possible to reduce risk perception biases (Weinstein, 1983). However, these efforts have taken place without having conducted the essential longitudinal studies. Such studies would take a large sample of young adolescents before they began to engage in risky behaviors, and then follow them long enough to observe their perceptions of risk over time, as they engage in the behaviors and possibly experience negative outcomes. It would be most desirable to see such studies conducted in populations representing different cultural backgrounds and levels of economic advantage. In addition to addressing some of the fundamental questions concerning the developmental trajectory of perceptions of risk and vulnerability, longitudinal studies also could inform us about some of their hypothesized developmental correlates such as future perspective, perspective taking, autonomy needs, and impulse control.

If risk judgments play a prominent role in the onset, continuation, or cessation of risky behavior, then perceptions about risk should continue to be incorporated into programs trying to prevent adolescent risk behavior and/or increase strategies to prevent such harm. Of course, doing so presents some real challenges. The actual risks posed by many of the behaviors we caution against are relatively small. Yet few educators would suggest providing adolescents with information about the actual risks, as doing so would (one fears) lead adolescents to minimize their importance. On the other hand, continuing to emphasize the likelihood of negative outcomes seems counterproductive if young people already feel a sense of heightened vulnerability, particularly in view of the inhibiting effects of excessive anxiety on preventive health behaviors (Leventhal, 1971). Furthermore, we have suggested that such an emphasis may backfire as adolescents become aware of the reality that most experiences with risky behaviors do not lead to negative outcomes and are in fact experienced as positive. A more appropriate goal in educating youth about health risks may be to find ways to translate small probabilities into real possibilities, without raising anxiety to unproductive levels.

Theoretical models can help inform us about potentially useful approaches to intervention, whether or not perceptions of risk prove to be crucial. For example, the Theory of Reasoned Action (Fishbein and Ajzen, 1975) includes a role for beliefs about the value attached to potential outcomes, expectations about social norms, and perceived benefits.

Programs that attempt to personalize and make vivid the reality of negative outcomes, such as those that expose adolescents to individuals who have AIDS, emphasize the meaning and impact of the outcomes rather than the probability of their occurrence (Sutton, 1982). To further develop such an emphasis would require not only that we understand what adolescents value, but also whether we, as a society, are providing adolescents with access to those outcomes. For many adolescents, such access is severely limited as a result of living in impoverished, racist, or violent environments. An even more challenging task would be to create opportunities that youth would find highly desirable, and which are simultaneously incompatible with risky behavior (Leventhal and Keeshan, 1993). Learning more about adolescents' perceptions of the benefits associated with engaging in risky behaviors could help in this endeavor. Perceived benefits typically are not studied, perhaps because of adults' understandable reluctance to acknowledge those benefits. Yet by helping us to understand better what draws adolescents to risky behavior, such research could assist us in identifying desirable alternatives to those behaviors.

The social normative component has been utilized in preventive interventions that attempt to correct adolescents' misperceptions about the number of teens engaging in risky behaviors. Adolescents who perceive higher levels of risk behavior in their peers view the risks of those behaviors as lower (Urberg and Robbins, 1984), and perceptions that peers condone more (or less) risky behavior are associated with more (or less) engagement in these behaviors (Boyer et al., 2000; DiClemente, 1991; Kinsman et al., 1998; Romer et al., 1994). Given that adolescents spend approximately twice as much time with their peers as they spend with parents or other adults (Brown, 1990; Savin-Williams and Berndt, 1990), peers and perceived peer norms thus become a major source of socialization and development during this period and a potentially effective intervention tool.

Understanding the relationship between risk judgment and behavior also will require that we turn attention to contextual factors that may influence the relationship. We tend to ask whether risk judgment influences behavior, rather than asking about the conditions under which it does (or does not). A person may agree that driving drunk is risky, but may decide to do so when under the influence of alcohol. Judgments concerning the risks of HIV may do little to influence the sexual behavior of someone who believes he or she will not live past the age of 30. These kinds of contextual factors are crucial but have received little attention. An example of a neglected and potentially important contextual factor is emotion. Emotion is known to influence adults' perceptions of risk (Isen, 1993; Nygren et al., 1996) as well as their risk tolerance. We would expect emotional states to influence adolescents' perceptions as well. Important questions include: How do specific emotions influence adolescents' judgments of risk? Do the effects of emotion on risk perception differ for adolescents and adults or as a function of development? For example, does fear play a more important role in adults' risk judgments than for adolescents'? In a given situation, do we see developmental differences in the degree to which emotion is experienced? To the degree that emotion is important, it would also have implications for the ways in which we study risk perception, suggesting that we create study environments that mimic the kinds of emotionally arousing situations in which judgments about risk are typically made.

The importance of risk perceptions—theoretically, in program development, and in defining standards of decision-making competence—warrants rigorous study. Existing literature is fraught with problems, primarily stemming from issues concerning the measurement of risk perceptions and from the lack of longitudinal studies. But the problems we have identified are solvable, and we are optimistic that future studies will be able to answer many of the pressing questions we have raised.

REFERENCES

Ajzen, I. (1985). From intentions to actions: A theory of planned behavior. In J. Kuhl & J. Beckman (Eds.), *Control: From cognition to behaviors* (pp. 11-39). New York: Springer-Verlag.

Alexander, C. S. (1989). Gender differences in adolescent health concerns and self-assessed health. *Journal of Early Adolescence, 9,* 467-479.

Ambuel, B. (1992). Social policy of adolescent abortion. *The Child, Youth, and Family Services Quarterly, 15*(2), 5-9.

American Cancer Society. (1979). *A study of health-related awareness and concerns among 4th, 5th and 6th graders (C.R.S. No. 5649).* New York: Author.

American School Health Association, Association for the Advancement of Health Education, & Society for Publication Health Education, Inc. (1989). *The national adolescent student health survey: A report on the health of America's youth.* Oakland, CA: Third Party.

Bachman, J. G. (1983). Schooling as a credential: Some suggestions for change. *International Review of Applied Psychology, 32*(4), 347-360.

Bandura, A. (1994). Social cognitive theory and exercise of control over HIV infection. In R. J. DiClemente & J. L. Peterson (Eds.), *Preventing AIDS: Theories and methods of behavioral interventions* (pp. 25-59). New York: Plenum Press.

Baron, R. M. (1988). An ecological framework for establishing a dual-mode theory of social knowing. In D. Bar-Tal & A. W. Kruglanski (Eds.), *The social psychology of knowledge* (pp. 48-82). Cambridge, England: Cambridge University Press.

Benedict, V., Lundeen, K. W., & Morr, B. D. (1981). Self-assessment by adolescents of their health status and perceived health needs. *Health Values: Achieving High Level Wellness, 5,* 239-245.

Benthin, A., Slovic, P., & Severson, H. (1993). Psychometric study of adolescent risk perception. *Journal of Adolescence, 16,* 153-168.

Bernstein, E., & Woodall, W. G. (1987). Changing perceptions of riskiness in drinking, drugs and driving: An emergency department-based alcohol and substance abuse prevention program. *Annals of Emergency Medicine, 16,* 1350-1354.

Beyth-Marom, R., Austin, L., Fischhoff, B., Palmgren, C., & Jacobs-Quadrel, M. (1993). Perceived consequences of risky behaviors: Adults and adolescents. *Developmental Psychology, 29*(3), 549-563.

Biehl, M., & Halpern-Felsher, B. L. (2001). Adolescents' and adults' understanding of probability expressions. *Journal of Adolescent Health, 28,* 30-35.

Bloom-Feshbach, S., Bloom-Feshbach, J., & Heller, K. A. (1982). Work, family, and children's perceptions of the world. In S. B. Kamerman & C. D. Hayes (Eds.), *Families that work: Children in a changing world* (pp. 268-307). Washington, DC: National Academy Press.

Boyer, C. B., Shafer, M. A., Wibbelsman, C. J., Seeberg, D., Teitle, E., & Lovell, N. (2000). Associations of sociodemographic, psychosocial, and behavioral factors with sexual risk and sexually transmitted diseases in teen clinic patients. *Journal of Adolescent Health, 27,* 102-111.

Brown, B. B. (1990). Peer groups and peer cultures. In S. S. Feldman & G. R. Elliott (Eds.), *At the threshold: The developing adolescent* (pp. 171-196). Cambridge, MA: Harvard University Press.

Brunswick, A. F. (1969). Health needs of adolescence: How the adolescent sees them. *American Journal of Public Health, 59,* 1730-1745.

Brunswick, A. F., & Josephson, E. (1972). Adolescent health in Harlem. *American Journal of Public Health, 62*(2) (Suppl. 2), 1-62.

Butterfield, F. (1996, May 12). States revamping laws on juveniles as felonies soar. *The New York Times,* p. 1.

Byler, R., Lewis, G. M., & Totman, R. J. (1969). *Teach us what we want to know.* New York, NY: Mental Health Materials Center.

Byrnes, J., Miller, D. C., & Reynolds, M. (1999). Learning to make good decisions: A self-regulation perspective. *Child Development, 70*(5), 1121-1140.

Centers for Disease Control and Prevention (1998). Youth risk behavior surveillance—United States, 1997. *Morbidity and Mortality Weekly Report (MMWR), 47*(SS-3).

Christiansen, B., Roehling, P., Smith, G., & Goldman, M. (1989). Using alcohol expectancies to predict adolescent drinking behavior after one year. *Journal of Consulting and Clinical Psychology, 57*(1), 93-99.

Cohn, L., Macfarlane, S., Yanez, C., & Imai, W. (1995). Risk-perception: Differences between adolescents and adults. *Health Psychology, 14*(3), 217-222.

Connell, J. P., & Halpern-Felsher, B. L. (1997). How neighborhoods affect educational outcomes in middle childhood and adolescence: Conceptual issues and an empirical example. In G. D. J. Brooks-Gunn & J. L. Aber (Eds.), *Neighborhood poverty Volume I: Context and consequences for children* (pp. 174-199). New York, NY: Russell Sage Foundation.

Covington, M. V., & Omelich, C. L. (1992). Perceived costs and benefits of cigarette smoking among adolescents: Need instrumentality, self-anger, and anxiety factors. In D. G. Forgays & D. K. Forgays (Eds.), *Anxiety: Recent developments in cognitive, psychophysiological, and health research* (pp. 245-261). Washington, DC: Hemisphere.

Davidson, A. R. (1995). From attitudes to actions to attitude change: The effects of amount and accuracy of information. In R. E. Petty and J. A. Krosnick (Eds.), *Attitude strength: Antecedents and consequences* (pp. 315-336). Mahwah, NJ: Lawrence Erlbaum Associates.

DiClemente, R. J. (1991). Predictors of HIV-preventive sexual behavior in a high-risk adolescent population: The influence of perceived peer norms and sexual communication on incarcerated adolescents' consistent use of condoms. *Journal of Adolescent Health, 12,* 385-390.

DiClemente, R. J., Zorn, J., & Temoshok, L. (1987). The association of gender, ethnicity, and length of residence in the Bay area to adolescents' knowledge and attitudes about Acquired Immune Deficiency Syndrome. *Journal of Applied Social Psychology, 17*(3), 216-230.

Drottz-Sjoberg, B.-M., & Sjoberg, L. (1991). Adolescents' attitudes to nuclear power and radioactive wastes. *Journal of Applied Social Psychology, 21,* 2007-2036.

Ebbesen, E. B., & Konecni, V. J. (1980). On the external validity of decision-making research: What do we know about decisions in the real world? In T.S. Wallsten (Ed.), *Cognitive processes in choice and decision behavior* (pp. 21-45). Hillsdale, NJ: Lawrence Erlbaum Associates.

Ellen, J. M., Adler, N. E., Dunlop, M. B., Gurvey, J. E., Millstein, S. G., & Tschann, J. M. (1998). Perceived risk for STDs and partner-specific condom intentions. *Pediatric Research, 43,* 4A.

Eme, R., Maisiak, R., & Goodale, W. (1979). Seriousness of adolescent problems. *Adolescence, 14*(53), 93-99.

Ey, S., Klesges, L. M., Patterson, S. M., Hadley, W., Barnard, M., & Alpert, B. S. (2000). Racial differences in adolescents' perceived vulnerability to disease and injury. *Journal of Behavioral Medicine, 23*(5), 421-435.

Federal Interagency Forum on Child and Family Statistics (2000). *America's children: Key national indicators of well-being.* Washington, DC: Author.

Feldman, W., Hodgson, C., Corber, S., & Quinn, A. (1986). Health concerns and health-related behaviours of adolescents. *Canadian Medical Association Journal, 134*(5), 489-493.

Ferguson, S. A., & Williams, A. F. (1996). Parents' views of driver licensing practices in the United States. *Journal of Safety Research, 27(2),* 171-180.

Finn, P., & Brown, J. (1981). Risks entailed in teenage intoxication as perceived by junior and senior high school students. *Journal of Youth and Adolescence, 10*(1), 61-76.

Fischhoff, B. (1996). The real world: What good is it? *Organizational Behavior and Human Decision Processes, 65,* 232-248.

Fischhoff, B., Parker, A. M., Bruine de Bruin, W., Downs, J., Palmgren, C., Dawes, R., & Manski, C. F. (2000). Teen expectations for significant life events. *Public Opinion Quarterly, 64,* 189-205.

Fishbein, M., & Ajzen, I. (1975). *Belief, attitude, intention, and behavior: An introduction to theory and research.* Reading, MA: Addison-Wesley.

Furby, L., Ochs, L. M., & Thomas, C. W. (1997). Sexually transmitted disease prevention: Adolescents' perceptions of possible side effects. *Adolescence, 32*(128), 781-809.

Gans, J. E., Alexander, B., Chu, R. C., & Elster, A. B. (1995). The cost of comprehensive preventive medical services for adolescents. *Archives of Pediatrics and Adolescent Medicine, 149*(11), 1226-1234.

Gerrard, M., Gibbons, F., Benthin, A., & Hessling, R. (1996a). A longitudinal study of the reciprocal nature of risk behaviors and cognitions in adolescents: What you do shapes what you think, and vice versa. *Health Psychology, 15*(5), 344-354.

Gerrard, M., Gibbons, F., & Bushman, B. (1996b). Relation between perceived vulnerability to HIV and precautionary sexual behavior. *Psychological Bulletin, 119*(3), 390-409.

Giblin, P. T., & Poland, M. L. (1985). Health needs of high school students in Detroit. *Journal of School Health, 55*(10), 407-410.

Gittler, J., Quigley-Rick, M., & Saks, M. J. (1990). *Adolescent health care decision making: The law and public policy.* Washington, DC: Carnegie Council on Adolescent Development.

Gladis, M., Michela, J., Walter, H., & Vaughan, R. (1992). High school students' perceptions of AIDS risk: Realistic appraisal or motivated denial? *Health Psychology, 11*(5), 307-316.

Gochman, D., & Saucier, J. F. (1982). Perceived vulnerability in children and adolescents. *Health Education Quarterly, 9*(2&3), 46/142-58/154.

Goldberg, J. H., Halpern-Felsher, B. L., & Millstein, S. G. (2001a). *Adolescent and adult errors in health risk judgments due to the representativeness heuristic.* Manuscript submitted for publication.

Goldberg, J. H., Halpern-Felsher, B. L., & Millstein, S. G. (2001b). *Beyond invulnerability: The importance of benefits in adolescents' decision to drink alcohol.* Manuscript submitted for publication.

Halpern-Felsher, B. L., & Cauffman, E. (2001). Costs and benefits of a decision: Decision-making competence in adolescents and adults. *Journal of Applied Developmental Psychology, 22,* 257-273.

Halpern-Felsher, B. L., Millstein, S. G., Ellen, J. M., Adler, N. E., Tschann, J. M., & Biehl, M. (2001). The role of behavioral experience in judging risks. *Health Psychology, 20,* 120-126.

Hamburg, D. A., Millstein, S. G., Mortimer, A. M., Nightingale, E. O., & Petersen, A. C. (1993). Adolescent health promotion in the twenty-first century: Current frontiers and future directions. In S. G. Millstein, A. C. Petersen, & E. O. Nightingale (Eds.), *Promoting the health of adolescents: New directions for the twenty-first century* (pp. 375-388). New York: Oxford University.

Hodne, C. J. (1995). Medical decision making. In M. W. O'Hara & R. C. Reiter (Eds.), *Psychological aspects of women's reproductive health* (pp. 267-290). New York: Springer.

Inhelder, B., & Piaget, J. (1958). *The growth of logical thinking from childhood to adolescence: An essay on the construction of formal operation structures.* New York: Basic Books.

Isen, A. M. (1993). Positive affect and decision making. In M. Lewis & J. M. Haviland (Eds.), *Handbook of emotions* (pp. 261-277). New York: Guilford Press.

Jacobs, J. E., & Potenza, M. (1991). The use of judgment heuristics to make social and object decisions: A developmental perspective. *Child Development, 62,* 166-178.

Kanfer, F. H. (1970). *Self regulation: Research, issues and speculations.* New York: Appleton-Century-Crofts.

Kaser-Boyd, N., Adelman, H. S., & Taylor, L. (1985). Minors' ability to identify risks and benefits of therapy. *Professional Psychology: Research & Practice, 16*(3), 411-417.

Kassinove, H., & Sukhodolsky, D. G. (1995). Optimism, pessimism and worry in Russian and American children and adolescents. *Journal of Social Behavior and Personality, 10*(1), 157-168.

Kinsman, S. B., Romer, D., Furstenberg, F. F., & Schwarz, D. F. (1998). Early sexual initiation: The role of peer norms. *Pediatrics, 102,* 1185-1192.

Klaczynski, P. A., & Narasimham, G. (1998). Representations as mediators of adolescent deductive reasoning. *Developmental Psychology, 34*(5), 865-881.

Kuhn, D. (1992). Thinking as an argument. *Harvard Educational Review, 62*(2), 155-178.

Kuhn, D., Amsel, E., O'Loughlin, M., Schauble, L., Leadbeater, B., & Yotive, W. (1988). *The development of scientific thinking skills.* San Diego, CA: Academic Press.

Leventhal, H. (1971). Fear appeals and persuasions: The differentiation of a motivational construct. *American Journal of Public Health, 61,* 1208-1224.

Leventhal, H., & Keeshan, P. (1993). Promoting healthy alternatives to substance abuse. In S. G. Millstein, A. C. Petersen, & E. O. Nightingale (Eds.), *Promoting the health of adolescents: New directions for the twenty-first century* (pp. 260-284). New York: Oxford University Press.

Lewis, C. C. (1980). A comparison of minors' and adults' pregnancy decisions. *American Journal of Orthopsychiatry, 50,* 446-453.

Lewis, C. C. (1981). How adolescents approach decisions: Changes over grades seven to twelve and policy implications. *Child Development, 52,* 538-544.

Manning, D. T., & Balson, P. M. (1989). Teenagers' beliefs about AIDS education and physicians perceptions about them. *Journal of Family Practice, 29,* 173-177.

Marks, A., Malizio, J., Hoch, J., Brody, R., & Fisher, M. (1983). Assessment of health needs and willingness to utilize health care resources of adolescents in a suburban population. *Journal of Pediatrics, 102*(3), 456-460.

McClure-Martinez, K., & Cohn, L. D. (1996). Adolescent and adult mothers' perceptions of hazardous situations for their children. *Journal of Adolescent Health, 18*(3), 227-231.

McKenna, F. P., Warburton, D. M., & Winwood, M. (1993). Exploring the limits of optimism: The case of smokers' decision making. *Bristish Journal of Psychology, 84,* 389-394.

Michielutte, R., & Diseker, R. (1982). Children's perceptions of cancer in comparison to other chronic illnesses. *Journal of Chronic Diseases, 35,* 843-852.

Midgley, C., & Feldlaufer, H. (1987). Students' and teachers' decision-making fit before and after the transition to junior high school. *Journal of Early Adolescence, 7*(2), 225-241.

Millstein, S. G., & Halpern-Felsher, B. L. (2001). *Judgments about risk and perceived invulnerability in adolescents and young adults.* Manuscript submitted for publication.

Millstein, S. G., & Irwin, C. E., Jr. (1985). Adolescents' assessments of behavioral risk: Sex differences and maturation effects. *Pediatric Research, 19,* 112A.

Moore, S., & Rosenthal, D. (1991). Adolescent invulnerability and perceptions of AIDS risk. *Journal of Adolescent Research, 6*(2), 164-180.

Moore, S., & Rosenthal, D. (1992). Australian adolescents' perceptions of health-related risks. *Journal of Adolescent Research, 7*(2), 177-191.

Mundt, J. C., Ross, L. E., & Harrington, H. L. (1992). A modeling analysis of young drivers' judgments of accident risk due to alcohol use and other driving conditions. *Journal of Studies on Alcohol, 53*(3), 239-248.

Natapoff, J. N., & Essoka, G. C. (1989). Handicapped and able-bodied children's ideas of health. *Journal of School Health, 59*(10), 436-440.

Nygren, T. E., Isen, A. M., Taylor, P. J., & Dulin, J. (1996). The influence of positive affect on the decision rule in risk situations: Focus on outcome (and especially avoidance of loss) rather than probability. *Organizational Behavior & Human Decision Processes, 66*(1), 59-72.

Office of Disease Prevention and Health Promotion. (1993). Recent reports on high-risk adolescents. *Public Health Reports, 108,* 68-77.

Parcel, G. S., Nader, P., & Meyer, M. (1977). Adolescent health concerns, problems, and patterns of utilization in a triethnic urban population. *Pediatrics, 60*(2), 157-164.

Parsons, J. T., Siegel, A. W., & Cousins, J. H. (1997). Late adolescent risk-taking: Effects of perceived benefits and perceived risks on behavioral intentions and behavioral change. *Journal of Adolescence, 20,* 381-392.

Piaget, J. (1971). The theory of stages in cognitive development. In D. R. Green, M. P. Ford, & G. B. Flamer, (Eds.), *Measurement and Piaget* (pp. 1-11). New York: McGraw-Hill.

Pleck, J. H., Sonenstein, F. L., & Ku, L. C. (1990). Contraceptive attitudes and intention to use condoms in sexually experienced and inexperienced adolescent males. *Journal of Family Issues, 11*(3), 294-312.

Pleck, J. H., Sonenstein, F. L., & Ku, L. C. (1993). Masculinity ideology: Its impact on adolescent males' heterosexual relationships. *Journal of Social Issues, 49*(3), 11-29.

Porteous, M. A. (1979). A survey of the problems of normal 15-year-olds. *Journal of Adolescence, 2,* 307-323.

Price, J. H., Desmond, S., & Kukulka, G. (1985). High school students' perceptions and misperceptions of AIDS. *Journal of School Health, 55*(3), 107-109.

Price, J. H., Desmond, S. M., Wallace, M., Smith, D., & Stewart, P. (1988). Differences on black and white adolescents' perceptions about cancer. *Journal of School Health, 58*(2), 66-70.

Quadrel, M. J., Fischhoff, B., & Davis, W. (1993). Adolescent (in)vulnerability. *American Psychologist, 48*(2), 102-116.

Radius, S. M., Dillman, T. E., Becker, M. H., Rosenstock, I., & Horvath, W. J. (1980). Adolescent perspectives on health and illness. *Adolescence, 25*(58), 375-384.

Reyna, V. F., & Ellis, S. C. (1994). Fuzzy-trace theory and framing effects in children's risky decision making. *American Psychological Society, 5*(5), 275-279.

Roe-Berning, S., & Straker, G. (1997). The association between illusions of invulnerability and exposure to trauma. *Journal of Traumatic Stress, 10*(2), 319-327.

Romer, D., Black, M., Ricardo, I., & Feigelman, S. (1994). Social influences on the sexual behavior of youth at risk for HIV exposure. *American Journal of Public Health, 84,* 977-985.

Ronis, D. L. (1992). Conditional health threats: Health beliefs, decisions, and behaviors among adults. *Health Psychology, 11*(2), 127-134.

Rosenstock, I. M. (1974). Historical origins of the Health Belief Model. *Health Education Monographs, 2,* 1-9.

Sastre, M. T. M., Mullet, E., & Sorum, P. C. (1999). Relationship between cigarette dose and perceived risk of lung cancer. *Preventive Medicine: An International Journal Devoted to Practice & Theory, 28*(6), 566-571.

Savin-Williams, R. C., & Berndt, T. J. (1990). Friendship and peer relations. In S. S. Feldman & G. R. Elliott (Eds.), *At the threshold: The developing adolescent* (pp. 277-307). Cambridge, MA: Harvard University Press.

Shaklee, H., & Goldston, D. (1989). Development in causal reasoning: Information sampling and judgment rule. *Cognitive Development, 4,* 269-281.

Smith, G., Goldman, M., Greenbaum, P., & Christiansen, B. (1995). Expectancy for social facilitation from drinking: The divergent paths of high-expectancy and low-expectancy adolescents. *Journal of Abnormal Psychology, 104*(1), 32-40.

Sobal, J., Klein, H., Graham, D., & Black, J. (1988). Health concerns of high school students and teachers' beliefs about student health concerns. *Pediatrics, 81*(2), 218-223.

Steinberg, L., & Silverberg, S. (1986). The vicissitudes of autonomy in early adolescence. *Child Development, 57,* 841-851.

Sternlieb, J. J., & Munan, L. (1972). A survey of health problems, practices, and needs of youth. *Pediatrics, 49*(2), 177-186.

Strunin, L. (1991). Adolescents' perceptions of risk for HIV infection: Implications for future research. *Social Science & Medicine, 32*(2), 221-228.

Sutton, S. R. (1982). Fear arousing communications: A critical examination of theory and research. In J. R. Eiser (Ed.), *Social psychology and behavioral medicine* (pp. 303-337). New York: John Wiley.

Triandis, H. C. (1977). *Interpersonal behavior.* Monterey, CA: Brooks Cole.

University of Minnesota. (1989). *The state of adolescent health in Minnesota.* Minneapolis: University of Minnesota Press.

Urberg, K., & Robbins, R. L. (1981). Adolescents' perceptions of the costs and benefits associated with cigarette smoking: Sex differences and peer influence. *Journal of Youth and Adolescence, 10*(5), 353-361.

Urberg, K., & Robbins, R. L. (1984). Perceived vulnerability in adolescents to the health consequences of cigarette smoking. *Preventive Medicine, 13,* 367-376.

Van der Plight, J. (1998). Perceived risk and vulnerability as predictors of precautionary behaviour. *British Journal of Health Psychology, 3,* 1-14.

Van der Velde, F. W., Hooykaas, C., & Van der Plight, J. (1996). Conditional versus unconditional risk estimated in models of AIDS-related risk behavior. *Psychology and Health, 12,* 87-100

Violato, C., & Holden, W. B. (1988). A confirmatory factor analysis of a four-factor model of adolescent concerns. *Journal of Youth & Adolescence, 17*(1), 101-113.

Weinstein, M. C., & Fineberg, H. (1980). *Clinical decision analysis.* Philadelphia, PA: Saunders.

Weinstein, N. (1980). Unrealistic optimism about future life events. *Journal of Personality and Social Psychology, 39*(5), 806-820.

Weinstein, N. D. (1983). Reducing unrealistic optimism about illness susceptibility. *Health Psychology, 2*(1), 11-20.

Weinstein, N. D. (1984). Why it won't happen to me: Perceptions of risk factors and susceptibility. *Health Psychology, 3*(5), 431-457.

Weinstein, N. D. (1989). Effects of personal experience on self-protective behavior. *Psychological Bulletin, 105*(1), 31-50.

Weithorn, L. A., & Campbell, S. B. (1982). The competency of children and adolescents to make informed treatment decisions. *Child Development, 53,* 1589-1598.

Whalen, C. K., Henker, B., O'Neil, R., Hollingshead, J., Holman, A., & Moore, B. (1994). Optimism in children's judgments of health and environmental risks. *Health Psychology, 13*(4), 319-325.

3

Vulnerability, Risk, and Protection

Robert William Blum, Clea McNeely, and James Nonnemaker

THE ORIGINS OF VULNERABILITY

As the morbidities of youth have shifted from primarily biophysiologic and infectious to social and behavioral, our thinking has changed regarding etiologies. Historically, both medicine and public health have sought to identify the biologic factors and infectious agents that predispose young people to morbidity and death. With mapping of the human genome, our ability to identify genetic factors that create vulnerabilities to a range of life-threatening conditions has reached a heretofore incomprehensible level of sophistication and specification. Likewise, ever since cholera was traced to the Broad Street pump in London, infectious disease epidemiologists have traced disease first to invasive organisms and more recently to behaviors. Thus, over the past generation we have come to understand the link between cigarette smoking and lung cancer, dietary practices and heart disease, and a range of other associations between behavior and health outcomes.

In adolescent health, where more than 75 percent of all mortality is related predominantly to social and behavioral factors, there has been ex-

The authors gratefully acknowledge Ann S. Masten, Cheryl Perry, Linda H. Bearinger, Michael Resnick, and Mary Story for their contributions to the conceptual framework presented in Figure 3-2.

tensive research over the past generation that has strived to identify the behaviors that predispose to negative health status both in the short term (during the teenage years) and long term (in adulthood). This stream of research, as Jessor (1991) notes, integrates behavioral epidemiology and social psychology. Over the past 25 years, it first proposed various theoretical frameworks. More recently it has marshaled the empirical data that support our understanding of how behaviors are interrelated, the factors that influence health risk behavior participation, and the factors associated with avoiding the same behaviors.

One problem that has complicated the research is the lack of a commonly agreed-on language. Specifically, we use the concept of "risk" in two distinctly different ways. One refers to risk-taking behaviors (e.g., smoking, drinking and driving, and unprotected sexual intercourse), which in themselves predispose to negative health outcomes (though in themselves they are not synonymous with the negative health outcomes such as emphysema, vehicular injury, and sexually transmitted diseases). Concurrently, we refer to the "at-risk" adolescent, which in our society too often is code for demographic "disadvantage" (e.g., minority status, poverty, and single-parent families). "At risk" may also refer to other disadvantage. As Rutter (1993), Garmezy (1987), Werner and Smith (1982), and others have shown, disadvantage may be biologic (e.g., diabetes), genetic (e.g., Trisomy 21), familial (e.g., mental illness), social (e.g., violent neighborhoods), or peer related (e.g., antisocial behaviors).

For the current paper, we refer to "vulnerability" as an interactive process between the social contexts in which a young person lives and a set of underlying factors that, when present, place the young person "at risk" for negative outcomes (e.g., school failure, unanticipated pregnancy, injury). Factors predisposing to vulnerability may be biologic (e.g., chronic illness) or cognitive (e.g., how risk is assessed). Vulnerabilities may result from being reared in disadvantaged environments such as in substance-abusing families, abusive/violent environments, or families with mental illness, and it can result from individual characteristics such as aggressive temperament.

Counter balancing such vulnerabilities are the resources (Patterson et al., 1990), assets (Benson, 1997), protective factors (Blum, 1998), and resilience (Masten et al. 1999) that likewise arise from the individual, familial, and social environments in which a young person lives. For example, individual characteristics that repeatedly have been found to be protective include social skills, intelligence, and a belief in a higher power beyond oneself. Protective family characteristics include a caring parent, an authoritative parenting style, and smaller family size. Likewise, social environments associated with reduced risk include caring nonfamilial adults, collective self-efficacy, and neighborhood engagement. Thus, as a dynamic process one must consider concurrently the factors that predispose to vulnerability and those that protect or buffer a young person from harm.

Vulnerability and Resilience

As a conceptual model, vulnerability and resilience has captured the imagination of researchers and program planners over the past decade. As an interactive process between context and harm-inducing/harm-minimizing factors, this research questions why some who are reared under extremely adverse circumstances appear to live healthy and productive lives while others faced with what appears to be minimal challenges never appear to overcome the adversities experienced in early life. Resilience is not a trait or characteristic that some have and others do not; rather, it represents an interaction between the individual and the environment (Garmezy, 1991). It is "the capacity to recover and maintain adaptive behavior after insult" (Bandura, 1979). Resilience implies resistance to threat, not invincibility (Garmezy, 1991) or invulnerability (Garmezy, 1985). Cumulative risk can defeat the most resilient individual. Rutter (1993) notes that resilience is interactive with vulnerabilities; it is developmental in nature, stemming from biology and experiences earlier in life; and protective factors may operate in different ways at different stages of development.

The developmental research of the 1970s and 1980s initially explored discrete aspects of adolescent development: physiological, cognitive, social, and moral. There was a search to identify universal markers of development; however, it has become increasingly clear through the work of Bronfenbrenner (1977, 1986), Bandura (1979), Harter (1987), and others that development does not occur independent of environment. Rather, it represents the adaptation of the individual to the environments in which he or she lives. Within such an interactive model, not only does the individual adapt to the environment, but the environment positively or adversely impacts development (Sameroff and Chandler, 1975). So, too, organic damage (e.g., brain trauma, severe chronic illness) can impede the physiologic "self-righting" tendency (Sameroff and Chandler, 1975).

Bandura (1979) also reinforced the interactive process of competence, resilience, vulnerability, and development. He observed that behavior is shaped by rewards and punishments that occur in specific social milieus reflecting social values. In addition, imitation of others (social learning) influences both behavior and self-identity.

Bronfenbrenner (1977, 1986), Sameroff et al. (1987), Bandura (1979), and others viewed the process of development not as the inevitable unfolding of predetermined characteristics, but more as a social construction in which the self develops through an ongoing interaction between the individual and the social contexts and social groups with whom the individual interacts (Berger and Luckmann, 1966). It is this interaction that led Goffman (1959) to observe that culture influences adolescent development through shaping identity, self-perception, and the public presentation of self. Such are the forces that influence, for example, adolescent dress and language, which in turn influence one's perception of self.

Grotberg (1994) used Erikson's stages (1950) to show how the acquisition and completion of tasks at each stage in development are closely linked with resilience. She noted that the three major sources of resilience (or protective factors) are an external facilitative environment, intrapsychic strengths, and internal coping skills. These are the same elements necessary for developmentally appropriate stage achievement. For example, an environment of unconditional love is necessary for a child to achieve Erikson's stage of autonomy. The consequence is a sense of being valued, which results in positive self-esteem (Baumrind, 1989). Positive self-esteem is a characteristic of resilience which, Grotberg (1994) noted, leads in turn to empathy (recognizing emotion, perspective and role taking, and emotional responsiveness), prosocial behaviors (helping, sharing, generosity, and sympathy), and problem behavior avoidance.

The link among vulnerability, resilience, and development rests in their all being interactive processes that endure over time in the context of the environments in which a young person lives. From a developmental perspective, resilience is the capacity to successfully undertake the work of each successive developmental stage in the face of significant factors that predispose to vulnerability (Garmezy, 1991).

Problem Behavior Theory

As conceptualized by Jessor (1992), *risk behavior* (what others term *problem behavior*) constitutes various behaviors that jeopardize one or more elements of health or development. Whether the behavior is drinking, early sexual intercourse, or drug use, Jessor argues that these are neither random nor thrill-seeking but rather "functional, purposive, instrumental, and goal-directed." Whether or not young people accurately assess the risk inherent in any given behavior, problem behavior theory holds that the actual (or perceived) risk pales next to the developmental goals they advance (e.g., presenting oneself as more mature). Simply stated, beating the odds is not a consideration in adolescent risk taking.

A second tenet of problem behavior theory is that there is substantial individual covariation in risk behaviors among adolescents, and although the pattern may vary regionally, among different ethnic groups, and in different economic strata, there is substantial empirical support for this tenet. Thus, it is reasonable to argue that there are common factors that link these often disparate behaviors (e.g., cigarette smoking and early sexual intercourse). What underlies these behaviors—what Jessor (1992) refers to as the "web of causation"—has five domains: biology/genetics, social environment, perceived environment, personality, and other behavior (see Figure 3-1). Each of these domains has associated risk and protective factors. These factors exert both direct and indirect influences, as depicted in Figure 3-1.

This paper elaborates the ecological model described by Jessor to include six domains: individual, family, peers, school, immediate social environments, and macrolevel environments. Figure 3-2 presents the framework as it is related to childhood through adolescence. This model places peer, school, and family influences on the individual within broader community and macrolevel contexts. Each domain has been the subject of extensive research over the past 20 years; a set of factors associated with risk and protection repeatedly have been identified for each domain. The factors noted within each domain as being either risk or protective are based on a generation of empirical research. As can be seen, most factors with demonstrated protective capacity are not merely the converse of risk factors—yet, some are. Most protective factors constitute a unique set that intersect with each other and with risk factors to create a "risk/assets gradient" for individual young people (Masten et al., 1999). But where risk and protection models are static snapshots in time, the ecological model is dynamic. Behaviors that may or may not result from the predisposing factors in turn enter into the model as factors that influence future development and thus themselves become risk or protective factors.

Although extensive research shows the associations between risk and protective factors and the likelihood of a young person participating in health risk behaviors, much remains poorly understood. Specifically, be-

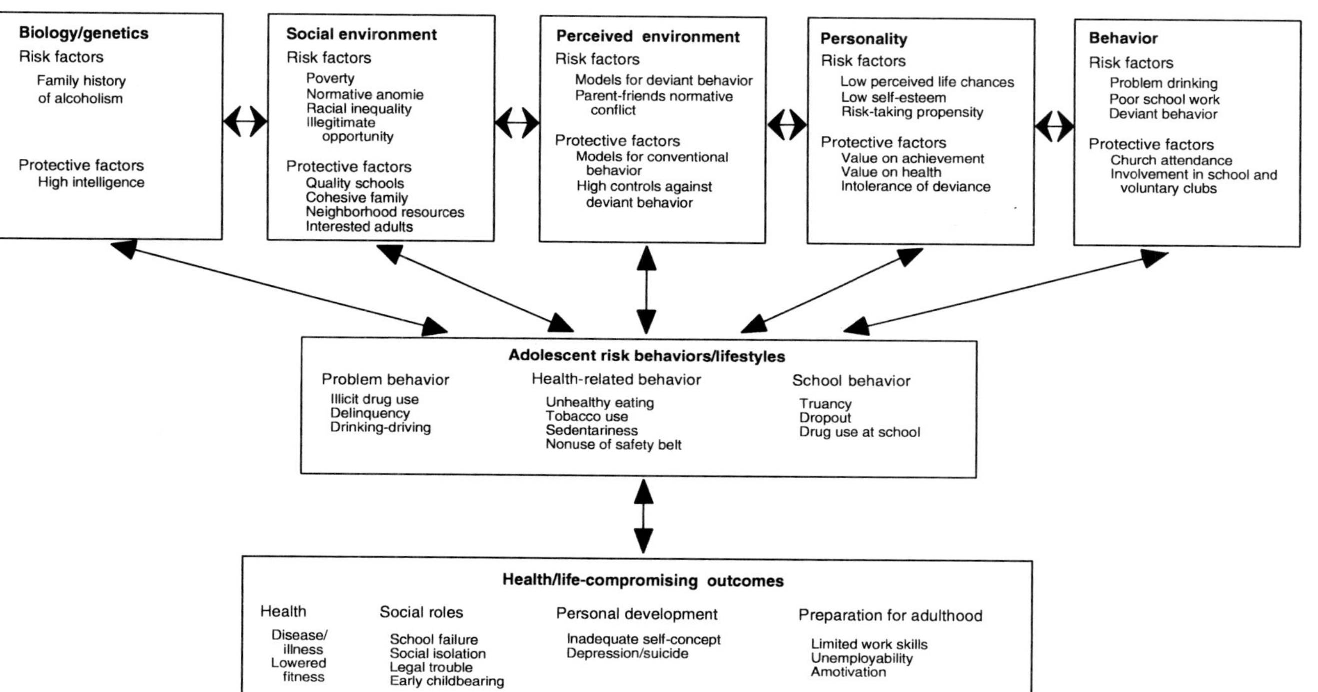

FIGURE 3-1 Interrelated conceptual domains of risk factors and protective factors.
SOURCE: Jessor (1992).

cause vulnerability is a process, how do protective factors work as buffers to diminish risk? Why are some factors protective or buffering for certain health risk behaviors (e.g., weapon-related violence) but not others (e.g., early onset of intercourse) despite the clustering of health-risk behaviors? These are the questions that are the subject of the subsequent section.

PROTECTIVE MECHANISMS AND VULNERABILITY

The level of vulnerability experienced by an individual or group of individuals (e.g., adolescents as a whole) can be described by the observed risk behaviors and outcomes. However, the *consequences* of a given level of vulnerability in either the short term or the long term cannot be predicted without also knowing the protective processes that operate to reduce the impact of risk/vulnerability.

Dozens of protective factors have been identified empirically (see Figure 3-2). We have less understanding, however, of how these protective factors work to diminish negative outcomes and/or promote positive ones (Jessor et al., 1998; Rutter, 1993). One reason protective mechanisms are not better delineated is their complexity. Building on the framework in Figure 3-2, this section of the paper presents three general propositions about how protective mechanisms may work to mitigate against negative health outcomes among adolescents.[1]

1. *Protective processes span multiple contexts.* Traditionally, research on risk and resiliency has identified protective mechanisms at the individual and the family levels. Additional protective mechanisms also operate at the environmental level (school, neighborhood, and peer group), and these macroprotective processes most likely condition the individual-level protective and risk mechanisms. For example, Sampson and colleagues (1997, 1999) found that individual adolescents were less likely to commit minor crimes in neighborhoods with high collective self-efficacy or in neighborhoods adjacent to those that had high collective self-efficacy. Although they did not test for cross-level interactions, it is possible that the potency of environmental protective factors such as collective self-efficacy depends

[1]We are not using the term protective processes as a synonym for resilience process. Resilience, by definition, operates when children are exposed to significant threat or severe adversity. Protective processes, however, operate for youth across a spectrum of risk.

on the accumulation of vulnerabilities and protective factors at the individual level. An environmental context may be protective for some individuals but increase vulnerabilities for others, depending on their individual-level attributes. For example, Werner and Smith (1992) found that military service promoted long-term work and family stability for young people whose academic plans did not extend beyond high school, but had the opposite effect on those whose plans included post-high school education.

2. *Protective processes vary across domains of functioning.* For example, a stimulating cognitive environment may promote intellectual development (Guo and Harris, 1999), but it is not necessarily protective for other outcomes such as early sexual intercourse.

3. *Protective processes vary across risk processes.* The same negative outcome can result from different risk processes. An individual or environmental characteristic may serve as a protective factor for one of those risk processes but not another. Hence a protective process may operate for only a subset of the adolescents "at risk" for a given outcome.

We illustrate the potential ways in which protective processes can function with an example. We select *school connectedness* to illustrate the pathways of protective influence because it is a protective factor that exerts a sizable effect on adolescent well-being and, in addition, is amenable to intervention. Resnick et al. (1997) found that when adolescents feel cared for by people at their school and feel like they are part of their school, they are less likely to use substances, engage in violence, or initiate sexual activity at an early age. Students who feel connected to school in this way also report higher levels of emotional well-being.

How does school connectedness protect adolescents from harm? Connection to caring adults is one of the key factors that promote healthy adolescent development (see, for example, Werner and Smith, 1992). In addition, students who are connected to school have greater access to school resources (e.g., extracurricular activities, individual investments by teachers, and opportunities with peers) than do their disengaged peers. In this regard, school connectedness operates as a form of social capital that allows students to make use of the human and financial capital schools have to invest in them. But how is school connectedness generated? We illustrate one pathway in this example.

Figure 3-3 illustrates a direct protective process. In this figure, the level of the individual protective factor (school connectedness) is determined, in

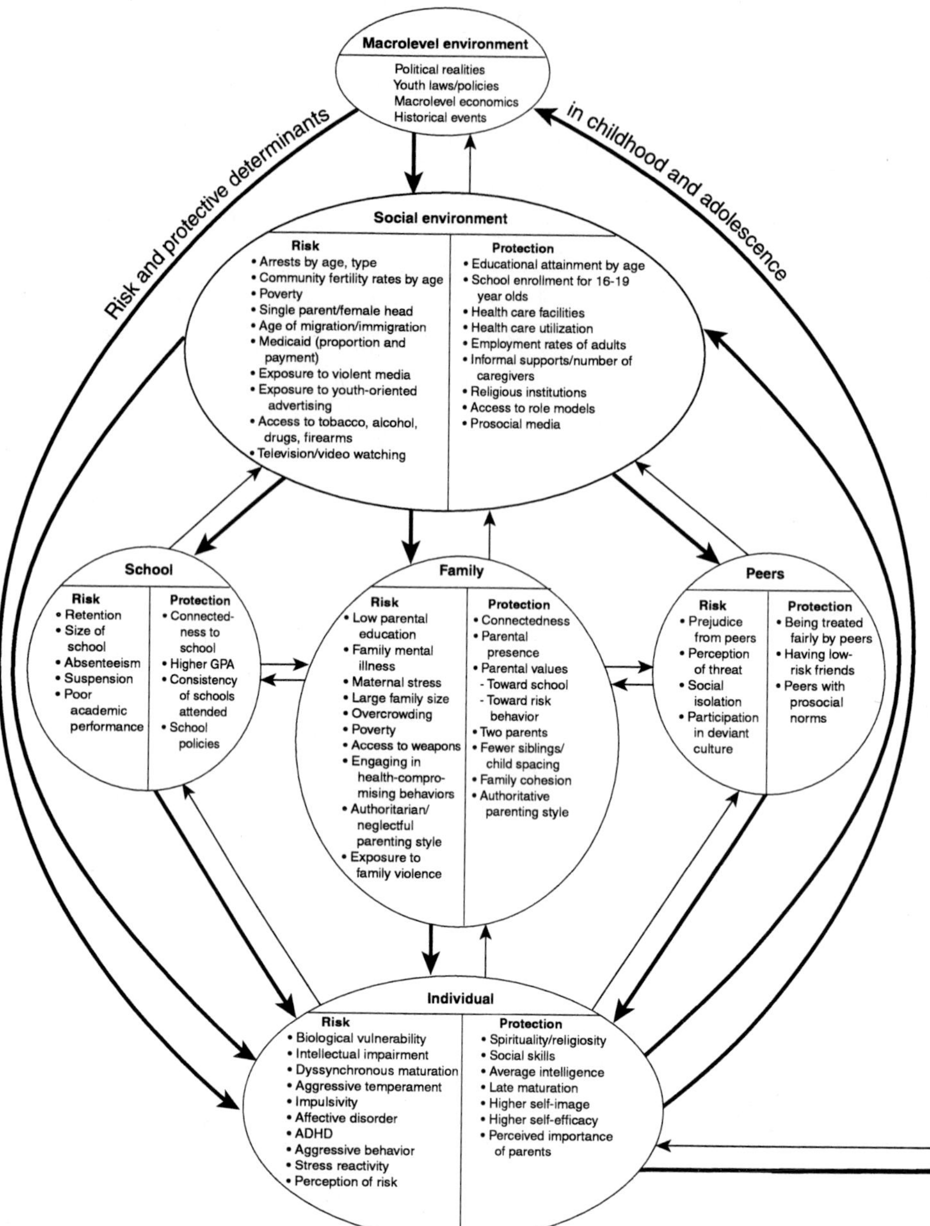

NOTE: The assignment of determinants as either risk or protective is not fixed as is implied in this model. Some factors may be protective depending on developmental stage or how terms are defined.

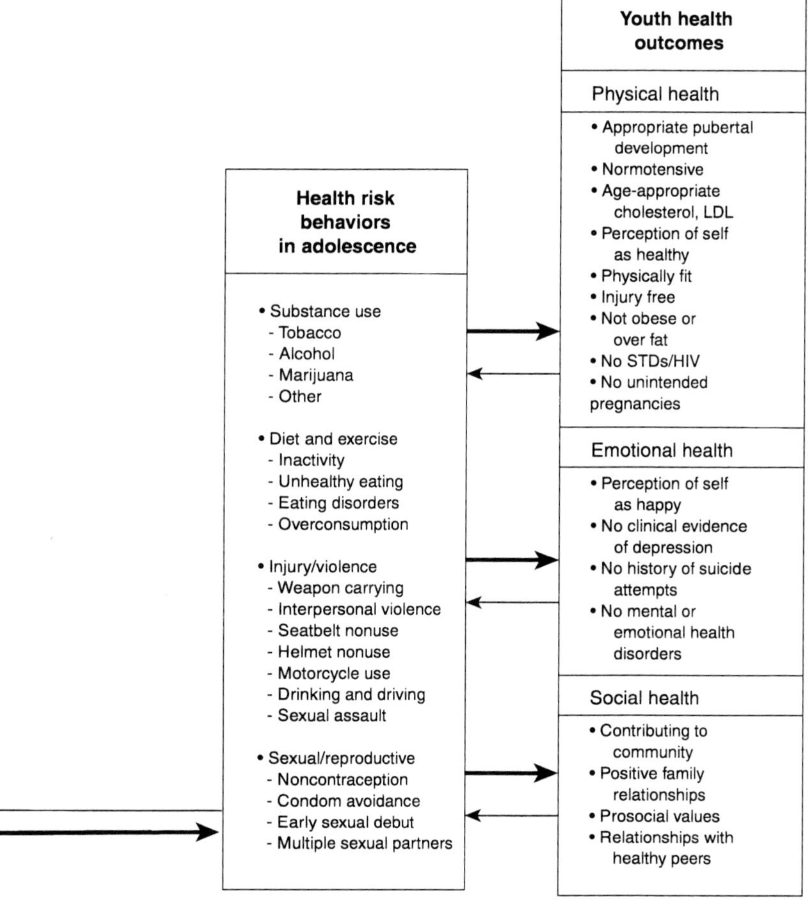

FIGURE 3-2 An ecological model of childhood antecedents of adolescent health risk behaviors and health outcomes.

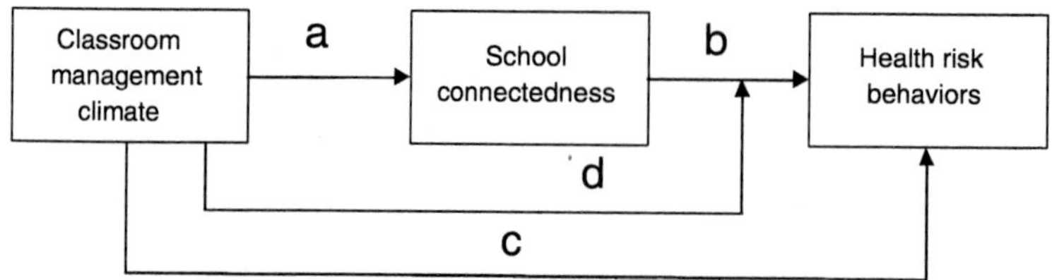

FIGURE 3-3 Direct protective process.
NOTE: See text for explanation of lettered arrows.

part, by the school environment. Specifically, students feel more connected to school when the school fosters a positive classroom management climate (McNeely et al., 2001). This is represented by the arrow marked "**a.**" School connectedness, in turn, directly affects the probability that adolescents will engage in health risk behaviors (pathway **b**).

It is also plausible that the classroom management climate has a direct effect on health risk behavior (e.g., violence) irrespective of the individual's school connectedness (see pathway **c**). Empirically the existence of pathway **c** would be supported by demonstrating that the association between the classroom management climate and the outcomes is not mediated entirely by school connectedness.

We also hypothesize that the nature of the direct protective process (pathway **b**) depends on the level of the school environmental variable. Put another way, the impact of the individual attributes is conditioned by the context within which they occur. For example, poorly managed classrooms (i.e., when students have trouble getting along with teachers, completing homework, and paying attention in class) may diminish the direct protective effect of connectedness because connected students in poorly managed classrooms have fewer resources to draw on than connected students in schools with positive classroom management climates. Conversely, in extremely well-managed classrooms, connectedness also may not be as highly protective because the direct effect of classroom management swamps the effect of connectedness. Alternatively, we might see an interaction such that good classroom management combined with high connectedness is an especially potent protective mechanism. These possibilities are represented by the arrow labeled **d.**

In the literature on risk and resiliency, protective factors traditionally have been defined as those that buffer or reduce the negative impact of the risk factor. This is illustrated by pathway **e** in Figure 3-4. In this example,

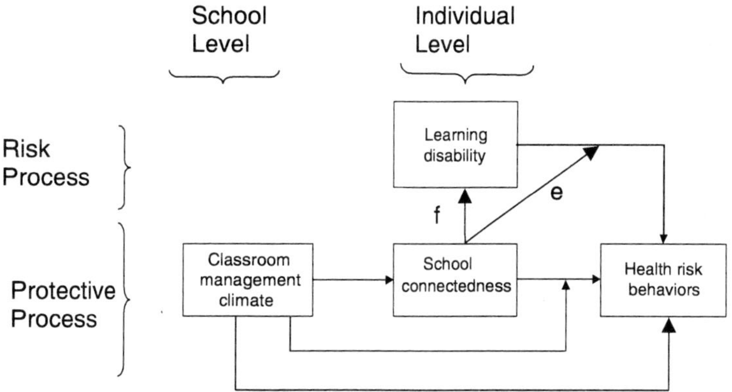

FIGURE 3-4 Protective buffering process.
NOTE: See text for explanation of lettered arrows.

low grade point average and having a learning disability are risk factors for negative health outcomes (Resnick et al., 1997). We select these risk factors for their reported association with multiple health risk behaviors.

Protective factors can buffer risk in two ways. The first possibility is that among students who feel highly connected to school, having a learning disability or a low grade point average confers no additional risk for the outcome because the protective process entirely wipes out the risk for the outcome generated by these vulnerabilities. Luthar et al. (2000) describe this type of effect modification as "protective-stabilizing." An alternative form of risk buffering is "protective but reactive." In this scenario, school connectedness buffers the risk generated by a learning disability or a low grade point average, but not completely.

In some cases, protective factors also can reduce or eliminate the risk factor directly, rather than simply mitigate the negative impact of the risk factor on the risky health behavior. This would be the case in our example if feeling highly connected to school *directly* helped a student improve his or her grade point average. This is illustrated by pathway **f.** Although not drawn in this figure nor tested empirically in the following text, it is important to note that risk buffering and risk reduction also can be generated directly by protective processes operating at the macro environment (school level).

In Figure 3-5, a causal relationship is hypothesized between the risk factor and school connectedness (connection **g**) such that having a low

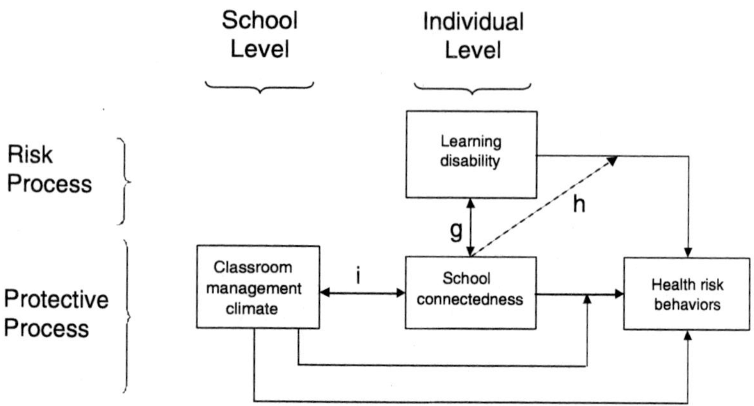

FIGURE 3-5 The risk process may deplete the protective process to the extent that buffering does not occur.
NOTE: See text for explanation of lettered arrows.

grade point average or a learning disability attenuates the individual's connection to school. This may happen to such an extent that the risk-buffering mechanism played by school connectedness in Figure 3-4 is overwhelmed by the risk. The dotted line of connection **h** indicates that the buffering mechanism no longer functions. This scenario is consistent with the argument in the vulnerability literature that in the face of overwhelming risk, all individuals will succumb to the risks in their environment. We are not suggesting, of course, that poor academic performance or a learning disability represent overwhelming risk. Determining the direction of the causal relationship between the risk factors and school connectedness requires longitudinal data.

Another bidirectional causal relationship is hypothesized between school connectedness and the classroom climate (connection **i**). Contextual effects generally are conceptualized as affecting individuals, and individuals are not granted the power in our models to affect their environment. However, in the case of schools, individual students can have a large impact on their environment, particularly a large negative impact. A common grievance of teachers is that one or two "bad apples" in the class disrupt the classroom and divert an inordinate amount of their time away from teaching. This bidirectional causal relationship also would require longitudinal data to test empirically.

We use the example laid out in Figures 3-3 through 3-5 and data from the National Longitudinal Study of Adolescent Health (Add Health) to empirically illustrate the three propositions at the beginning of this section: (1) protective processes span multiple contexts; (2) protective processes vary across domains of functioning; and (3) protective processes vary across risk processes.

Add Health is a nationally representative sample of in-school youth in grades 7–12 (for a description of the sample, see Resnick et al., 1997, and Bearman et al., 1997). The present empirical illustration uses data from the first wave (1995) in-home sample of 20,775 students and from the parent survey, which was conducted at the time of the in-home survey. The school-level protective factor and the school-level control variables are measured using data from the in-school survey of approximately 90,000 students.

We explore the risk and protective processes for three health risk behaviors: *ever had sex, ever used cocaine,* and *weapon-related violence.* Weapon-related violence is defined as having committed at least one of the following acts in the past year: threatened to use a weapon to get something from someone, pulled a knife or gun on someone, shot or stabbed someone, used a weapon in a fight, or hurt someone badly enough to need bandages or medical care. The three health risk behaviors often are considered as part of a problem behavior syndrome (Baumrind, 1989). Although they are correlated, we consider them separately to demonstrate that macro-level protective processes may differ, even across correlated outcomes. As shown in Table 3-1, 40 percent of the sample has had sex. Just 3 percent have ever tried cocaine. A disturbing number of adolescents—nearly a quarter of the sample—engaged in weapon-related violence or beat someone so badly they needed medical care in the past year.

In the present example, the two protective factors are individual-level *school connectedness* and the average *classroom management climate* in a school. School connectedness is a scale consisting of students' reports of how much they agree or disagree with six statements: you feel that your teachers care about you; you feel like you are part of your school; you feel close to people at your school; you are happy to be at your school; the teachers at your school treat students fairly; and you feel safe in your school. The scale has adequate reliability (α = .77) and ranges from 0 to 4. The mean level of school connectedness is 2.66, indicating that most students feel moderately connected to school.

The school-level classroom management climate is the school mean of responses to four questions in the in-school survey. Students were asked how much trouble they have getting along with their teachers, getting along

TABLE 3-1 Description of Health Risk Behaviors, Protective Factors, and Risk Factors

	Mean/ Proportion	S.D.	Minimum	Maximum	N
Health Risk Behaviors					
Weapon-related violence	.23		0	1	20,084
Ever had sexual intercourse	.40		0	1	20,009
Ever used cocaine	.03		0	1	19,826
Protective Factors					
School connectedness	2.66	.71	0	4.0	19,820
Classroom management climate	2.39	.19	1.8	3.9	19,533
Risk Factors					
GPA	2.76	.77	1.0	4.0	19,353
Learning disability	.16		0	1	17,231

SOURCE: Data from the National Longitudinal Study of Adolescent Health, Wave 1, see Bearman et al., 1997.
NOTES: Sample sizes vary due to missing data. All means are unweighted, and hence not necessarily nationally representative.

with other students, getting their homework done, and paying attention in class. Responses range from never to every day (0 to 4). The scale was reverse coded so that a higher value indicates a more positive classroom management climate. The classroom management scale has good reliability (α = .83). The schools in this sample have moderate problems with classroom management. The school-level average is 2.4, which equates roughly to each student in the classroom having trouble getting along, paying attention, or doing homework slightly less than once a week. The range across schools is 1.8 to 3.4 (out of a potential range of 0 to 4).

The two risk factors in the model are *grade point average* (GPA) and having a *learning disability*. The average self-reported GPA of students is 2.7. Learning disability is a dichotomous variable based on a parent's report of whether a son or daughter has a learning disability or is in a special education class. A respondent is coded as having a learning disability if his or her parent reports affirmatively to both of these questions.

All analyses include the following control variables: age, 2 years older than average age for grade, 2 years younger than average age for grade, gender, race/ethnicity, family income, family structure, urbanicity, ever suspended or expelled from school, individual-level classroom behavior (the individual score on the classroom management scale), and the following school characteristics: public (yes versus no), school size, percentage of two-parent families, percentage of African American, and percentage of African American squared.

Our modeling strategy proceeds in three steps. First, the effect of school-level classroom management on individual-level school connectedness is estimated using ordinary least squares regression (OLS) (Model 1 in Table 3-2). Second, the effect of both protective factors, and their interaction, on the health risk behaviors is estimated with a series of logit models (Models 2 through 4 in Table 3-2). Finally, the logit models are reestimated with the addition of the risk factors and their interaction with school connectedness (see Table 3-4 later in this text). All continuous variables in the models are centered, that is, the mean value of the variable is subtracted from each score. These analyses are cross-sectional and do not establish causality. The goal is to illustrate a range of protective mechanisms rather than to determine the actual strength of these protective factors.

Table 3-2 demonstrates that protective processes can span multiple contexts. Model 1 shows that the classroom management climate is positively associated with school connectedness: In positive classroom management climates, students report feeling slightly more connected to school. Hence the individual-level protective factor is a function, in part, of the school environment. Moreover, for one outcome—weapon-related violence—the school-level classroom management climate and individual-level school connectedness have independent effects. For two of the outcomes, the school-level protective factor conditions the direct effect of the individual-level protective factor.

Models 2 through 4 in Table 3-2 demonstrate the second proposition, that the protective process differs across outcomes, or domains of functioning. The classroom management climate *directly influences* weapon-related violence, but has no effect on students' decisions to initiate sexual intercourse or experiment with cocaine. The classroom management climate *moderates* the protective effect of school connectedness on weapon-related violence and sexual activity, such that school connectedness is a more potent protective factor when classroom management is high. In the case of sexual activity, classroom management moderates the protective effect of school connectedness, even though classroom management itself has no direct effect on the sexual activity.

TABLE 3-2 Protective Processes for Weapon-Related Violence, Ever Had Sexual Intercourse, and Ever Used Cocaine

	OLS Coefficients	Logistic Regression Coefficients		
	Model 1: School Connectedness	Model 2: Weapon-Related Violence	Model 3: Ever Had Intercourse	Model 4: Ever Used Cocaine
School connectedness		–.33* (.03)	–.34* (.03)	–.48* (.06)
Classroom management	.12* (.04)	-.42* (.16)	.20 (.25)	–.27 (.46)
School connectedness × classroom management		–.28* (.13)	–.40** (.14)	
χ^2 (d.f.)	n.a.	2617.09 (24)	2329.00 (24)	659.94 (24)
N	18,320	18,666	18,593	18,442

SOURCE: Data from the National Longitudinal Study of Adolescent Health, Wave 1, see Bearman et al., 1997.

NOTES: Standard errors in parentheses. All standard errors adjusted for the complex sampling design. All models are unweighted and include the following variables: age, 2 years older than average age for grade, 2 years younger than average age for grade, gender, race/ethnicity, family income, family structure, urbanicity, ever suspended or expelled from school, individual-level classroom behavior (the individual score on the classroom management scale), school sector (public versus else), school size, percentage of two-parent families, percentage African American, and percentage African American squared.

*p<.05. **p<.01.

The nature of the effect modification is illustrated in Table 3-3. The three columns present the effect of school connectedness on the health risk behaviors at the low, medium, and high levels of classroom management. The first row presents the odds ratios for violence. In the average school, the adjusted odds ratio associated with a one-unit increase in school connectedness is .72. (Because the variables are centered, this is simply the exponentiated coefficient for the main effect in Table 3-2, i.e., $e^{-.33}$.) In

TABLE 3-3 Effect of School Connectedness on Health Risk Behaviors at Different Levels of Classroom Management Climate, Odds Ratios, and 95 Percent Confidence Intervals

	Level of Classroom Management		
	1 S.D. Below Mean	Mean	1 S.D. Above Mean
Weapon-related violence	.76 (.68, .84)	.72 (.68, .78)	.68 (.60, .76)
Ever had intercourse	.76 (.79, .81)	.71 (.67, .75)	.66 (.61, .71)
Ever used cocaine	.61 (.55, .68)	.61 (.55, .68)	.61 (.55, .68)

SOURCE: Data from the National Longitudinal Study of Adolescent Health, Wave 1, see Bearman et al., 1997.

NOTES: Odds ratios and confidence intervals are calculated from models in Table 3-2 and standard deviations (S.D.) presented in Table 3-1. For example, the odds ratios for weapon-related violence were calculated as follows: One S.D. below the mean: $e^{(-.33+[-.28*-.19])}$; one S.D. above the mean: $e^{(-.33+[-.28*.19])}$.

*p<.05.

schools with positive classroom management climates (climates that are one standard deviation above the mean), the odds ratio is .68. In schools with poorly managed classrooms, however, the protective power of school connectedness declines. A similar pattern is evident for sexual activity. Because there is no effect modification for cocaine use, school connectedness is equally protective against cocaine use at all levels of classroom management.

Health risk behaviors cluster together. Adolescents often become involved in several health risk behaviors, rather than just one or two. Consequently, research and prevention strategies should target several health risk behaviors, as does the Burt et al. paper in this volume. However, the results in Table 3-2 also illustrate that whereas some protective processes operate for all or most health risk behaviors (e.g., school connectedness), others are specific to certain outcomes. In this example, the classroom management climate directly reduces weapon-related violence but does not directly influence other outcomes. The specificity of protective processes has implications for research and interventions. Some protective factors may be particularly powerful in that they not only directly influence adolescents' probability of engaging in risky behaviors, but they also make other protective factors more potent. These factors would be the ideal targets for inter-

TABLE 3-4 Protective Buffering Process for Weapon-Related Violence, Unweighted Logistic Regression Coefficients

	Model 1	Model 2
School connectedness	–.31***	–.31***
	(.04)	(.03)
Classroom management climate	–.35*	–.47**
	(.16)	(.16)
School connectedness × classroom management	–.26*	–.34**
	(.13)	(.13)
GPA	–.24***	
	(.03)	
GPA X school connectedness	–.09*	
	(.03)	
Learning disability		.17***
		(.06)
Learning disability × school connectedness		.00
		(.07)
χ^2 (d.f.)	2450.25 (25)	1287.15 (25)
N 18,225	16,325	

SOURCE: Data from the National Longitudinal Study of Adolescent Health, Wave 1, see Bearman et al., 1997.
NOTES: Standard errors in parentheses. All standard errors adjusted for the complex sampling design. Both models include full set of control variables. Odds ratios can be calculated as in Table 3-3. For example, the odds ratio for gpa among students with low school connectedness (one s.d. below the mean) is $e^{.24+(.09*-.71)}$. The odds ratio for gpa among students with high school connectedness (one s.d. above the mean) is $e^{.24+(.09*.71)}$.
*p<.05. **p<.01. ***p<.001.

vention. Other protective factors might be key to enhancing particular developmental outcomes but not others.

Table 3-4 demonstrates the third general proposition, that protective processes vary across risk factors. For simplicity we focus on a single outcome, weapon-related violence. We compare the protective buffering mechanisms across the two risk factors: having a learning disability and receiving low grades in school. Model 1 presents the direct effect of GPA on weapon-related violence, holding the other variables constant at their means. A one-point decrease in GPA is associated with an increased risk of participating in weapon-related violence of 27 percent ($e^{.24}-1$). Model 2 shows that having a learning disability is associated with an increased risk of 18 percent ($e^{.17} - 1$).

The risk factor-school connectedness interaction terms test for the presence of a protective buffering process. School connectedness *does not* moderate the risk engendered by having a learning disability (Model 2). In contrast, school connectedness *does* moderate the risk associated with a low GPA, but not in the manner expected (Model 1). If risk buffering were present, the association between GPA and weapon-related violence would be weakest at high levels of school connectedness and strongest at low levels of school connectedness. Instead, the opposite is true. Among students with low school connectedness (one standard deviation below the mean), a one-point decline in GPA is associated with a 19-percent increase in the risk of participating in weapon-related violence. In contrast, among students with high school connectedness (one standard deviation above the mean), a one-point decline in GPA is associated with a 35-percent increase in the risk of weapon-related violence.

The implication of this finding is that strategies to reduce violence by improving or maintaining GPA will be more effective in schools where students feel connected to school than in schools where students feel disconnected, even if the intervention strategy achieves similar gains in GPA in both types of schools. In practice, of course, successful programs to improve academic achievement also address students' connections to school. More broadly, the results in Table 3-4 illustrate that the risk environment must be taken into account when working to enhance protective processes. Likewise, the payoff to reducing risk will depend on the protective processes at play.

CONCLUSION

Over the past generation, our understanding of what predisposes young people to harm has shifted from viewing vulnerabilities as discrete, intrapsychic factors to seeing them as an interlocking set of factors that is heavily influenced by the contexts within which young people live. More recently we have come to understand the interrelationships between predisposing factors that create vulnerability and the countervailing forces that buffer, moderate, or alter the trajectory that otherwise leads to what Schorr (1997) refers to as "rotten outcomes."

This paper presents a model of understanding adolescent vulnerability processes across six interrelated domains—from the individual- to macro-level factors—and then tests three possible ways that protective factors alter risky health behaviors such as violence, cocaine use, and sexual intercourse. What is evident is that the relationships are complex and that the ways in which protective factors work differ across contexts and across outcomes. For example, in our illustration we found that the classroom management climate is a key protective factor for weapon-related violence: It has a direct protective effect; it promotes school connectedness, another protective factor; and it enhances the protective effect of school connectedness. In contrast, the classroom management climate does little to protect against cocaine use or sexual intercourse.

Teasing apart these relationships is not merely an academic exercise. It is important for policy and intervention. Traditionally, policy and intervention efforts focused on eliminating the factors that put young people in harm's way. More recently, with the understanding that it is essential to strengthen the protective factors in the lives of young people (in addition to reducing vulnerabilities), policies and programs have focused on building young people's assets. The models and illustrative examples in this paper highlight the importance of going beyond a simple accounting of vulnerabilities and protective factors. For a policy or intervention to be optimally effective, it must take into account how vulnerability and protective processes are linked. In the final analysis, our goal must be not only the avoidance of risk, but the achievement of maximal potential for each adolescent.

REFERENCES

Bandura, A. (1979). Self-efficacy: Toward a unifying theory of behavioral change. *Psychology Review, 84,* 191-215.

Baumrind, R. (1989). Rearing competent children. In W. Damon (Ed.), *Child development today and tomorrow: New direction in child development* (pp. 349-378). San Francisco: Jossey-Bass.

Bearman, P. S., Jones, J., & Udry, J. R. (1997). *The national longitudinal study of adolescent health: Research design.* Available: <http://www.cpc.unc.edu/addhealth>. [August 8, 2001].

Benson, P. (1997). *All kids are our kids.* San Francisco: Jossey-Bass.

Berger, P., & Luckmann, T. (1966). *The social construction of reality.* New York: Doubleday.

Blum, R. W. (1998). Healthy youth development as a model for youth health promotion: A review. *Journal of Adolescent Health, 22*(5), 368-375.

Bronfenbrenner, U. (1986). Ecology of the family as a context for human development: Research perspectives. *Developmental Psychology, 22*(6), 723-742.

Brofenbrenner U. (1977). Toward an Experimental Ecology of Human Development. *American Psychologist, 32,* 513-531.

Erikson, E. (1950). *Childhood and society.* New York: W. W. Norton.

Garmezy, N. (1987). Stress, competence, and development: Continuities in the study of schizophrenic adults, children vulnerable to psychopathology, and the search for stress-resistant children. *American Journal of Orthopsychiatry, 57,* 159-174.

Garmezy, N. (1991). Resiliency and vulnerability to adverse developmental outcomes associated with poverty. *American Behavioral Sciences, 34,* 416-430.

Goffman, E. (1959). *The presentation of self in everyday life.* New York: Doubleday.

Grotberg, E. (1994). *Promoting resilience in children: A new approach.* Birmingham: University of Alabama, The Civitan Center.

Guo, G., & Harris, K. M. (1999). The mechanisms mediating the effects of poverty on children's intellectual development. *Demography, 37,* 431-447.

Harter, S. (1987). The perceived competence scale for children. *Child Development, 33,* 87-97.

Jessor, R. (1991). Behavioral science: An emerging paradigm for social inquiry? In R. Jessor (Ed.), *Perspectives on behavioral science: The Colorado lectures* (pp. 309-316). Boulder, CO: Westview Press.

Jessor, R. (1992). Risk behavior in adolescence: A psychosocial framework for understanding and action. In D. E. Rogers and E. Ginzburg (Eds.), *Adolescents at risk: Medical and social perspectives* (pp. 19-34). Boulder, CO: Westview Press.

Jessor, R., Turbin, M. S., & Costa, F. (1998). Protective factors in adolescent health behavior. *Journal of Personality & Social Psychology, 75*(30), 788-800.

Luthar, S. S., Cicchetti, D., & Becker, B. (2000). The construct of resilience: A critical evaluation and guidelines for future work. *Child Development, 71,* 543-562.

Masten, A. S., Hubbard, J. J., Gest S. D., Tellegen, A. Garmezy, N., & Ramirez, M. (1999). Competence in the context of adversity: Pathways to resilience and maladaptation from childhood to late adolescence. *Development and Psychopathology, 11*(1), 143-169.

McNeely, C. S., Nonnemaker, J., & Blum, R. (2001). School connectedness: The untapped power of schools to diminish risk behaviors. Paper presented at the annual meeting of the American Sociological Association, Anaheim, CA, August 18-21.

Patterson, J., McCubbin, H., & Warwick, W. (1990). The impact of family functioning on health changes in children with cystic fibrosis. *Social Science and Medicine, 31*(2), 159-164.

Resnick, M., Bearman, P., Blum, R., Bauman, K. E., Harris, K. M., Jones, J., Tabor, J., Beuhring, T., Sieving, R. E., Shew, M., Ireland, M., Bearinger, L. H., & Udry, J. R. (1997). Protecting adolescents from harm: Findings from the National Longitudinal Study on Adolescent Health. *Journal of the American Medical Association, 278*(10), 823-832.

Rutter, M. (1993). Resilience: Some conceptual considerations. *Journal of Adolescent Health 14,* 626-631.

Sameroff, A., & Chandler, M. (1975). Reproductive risk and the continuum of caretaking causality. In F. Horowitz (Ed)., *Review of child development* (pp. 187-244). Chicago: University of Chicago Press.

Sameroff, A., Seifer, R., Barocas, R., Zax, M., & Greenspan, S. (1987). Intelligence quotient scores of 4-year-old children: Social-environmental risk factors. *Pediatrics, 79,* 343-350.

Sampson, R. J., Morenoff, J. D., & Earls, F. (1999). Beyond social capital: Spatial dynamics of collective efficacy for children. *American Sociological Review, 64,* 633-660.

Sampson, R. J., Raudenbush, S., & Earls, F. (1997). Neighborhoods and violent crime: A multilevel study of collective self-efficacy. *Science, 277,* 918-924.

Schorr, L. (1997). *Common purpose: Strengthening families and neighborhoods to rebuild America.* New York: Doubleday.

Werner, E., & Smith, R. (1982). *Vulnerable but invincible.* New York: McGraw-Hill.

Werner, E., & Smith, R. (1992). *Overcoming the odds.* New York: Cornell University Press.

4

Modeling the Payoffs of Interventions to Reduce Adolescent Vulnerability

Martha R. Burt, Janine M. Zweig, and John Roman

INTRODUCTION

Public policy often has been blind to adolescents, except when it has focused on aspects of their behavior that trouble their elders. Too often, policy makers limit their attention to artificially narrow and isolated aspects of youth behavior. They consider only health, or only criminal, or only educational issues. In addition, the payoff of youth vulnerability and our failure to ameliorate it are rarely addressed. The few existing treatments of the cost of adolescent risk behaviors have likewise focused on single behaviors (e.g., teen childbearing—Burt, 1985, 1986; Burt and Levy, 1987) or narrowly defined patterns (e.g., being a career criminal—Cohen, 1998). A just-released report identifying important future research issues related to youth (Millstein et al., 2000) does not even mention cost, either as the cost of outcomes to society or the cost of interventions or approaches to produce better outcomes. The absence of cost concerns is even more striking as Millstein and her colleagues review and summarize a decade of published documents that in their turn summarize and integrate research on adolescence and make recommendations for future research.

Compared to very young children and the elderly, adolescents suffer

---

Although the authors are affiliated with the Urban Institute, the views expressed in this chapter are those of the authors and should not be attributed to the Urban Institute, its trustees, or its funders.

from few conditions that will kill them while they are still young. The formation in adolescence of certain health habits with long-term negative consequences (such as smoking tobacco products, use of other addictive substances, or sexual activity without protection from STD and AIDS) often does not produce morbidity or mortality *in adolescence itself.* Rather the effects, and the payoffs, develop over a lifetime. Other behaviors such as school dropout, running away from home, or criminal involvement also exert their most powerful effects in adulthood. Thus, when societies face decisions about where to invest significant health and other supportive resources, programs for adolescents often receive short shrift. This is true despite the fact that after early infancy, adolescence is the period of greatest vulnerability, during which patterns and habits affecting a lifetime are established and solidified.

In 1998, youth made up about one in every seven people in the U.S. population, whether the focus is on the younger end of the age spectrum (10–19 year olds were 14.3 percent) or the older end (15–24 year olds were 13.8 percent). These are the individuals on whom the future of this country rides. A strong argument can be made that we need *all* of our youth to develop into productive adults, with skills and attitudes ready to cope with twenty-first-century work, politics, and community and interpersonal relationships. The evidence suggests that for significant portions of our youth, seriously inadequate educational achievement, and life-threatening habits such as addictions, risky sexual behavior, involvement in crime and violence, and too-early childbearing foreclose the possibility that they will become contributing members of society.

With respect to adolescents, the focus of attention is far too often on individual behavior, with far less attention being paid to context. But context is critical for understanding, and perhaps altering, the choices that youth make about their own behavior. For youth to make prosocial choices, it is essential that communities create increasingly broad and rewarding economic and social opportunities. There is an important interaction between economic opportunity and the readiness of today's youth to take advantage of it. Without the realistic hope of getting ahead economically, there is little incentive for youth to invest in education or refrain from some of the less healthy, or less legal, habits they may acquire during adolescence. But without the expectation that there will be a qualified workforce to fill newly created jobs, many employers will send jobs overseas or fill them with people trained outside the United States, while the jobs that remain will be the least challenging, interesting, and rewarding ones. To the extent that the youth of today and tomorrow are not prepared for the future (and many are not), expectations for the country's continued economic prosperity are open to question.

We have choices to make. We can invest society's resources in activities that will increase the odds that youth will become contributing members of society, or we can invest primarily in institutions such as health services or prisons designed only to compensate or protect society from the consequences of their negative behaviors. Given these choices, the payoffs from the former over the latter should make the policy choices clear. This paper is an exercise in designing an approach to illuminate the costs and opportunities of various policy choices with respect to investing in youth.

Why We Need to Think About Payoffs (Costs and Benefits)

Americans have a very strong belief in the efficacy of individual initiative and self-reliance. Far too often, and in too many arenas, this translates into policies that withhold support and investment in people until they fail, and then spend considerable sums on programs that try to protect society from the results or, on occasion, pick up the pieces. The earlier these policies are applied in people's lives, the more global the ultimate effects. Failing to invest in securing productive futures for this nation's most vulnerable youth has implications for everything from family formation to economic competitiveness. Yet public policy in this country related to people's well-being rarely issues from considerations of "the big picture." In part this is an inevitable aspect of how politics works in America, but in part it stems from lack of information, and information can sometimes make a difference to policy.

To give one example, at the request of the (then) Center for Population Options, a research and advocacy organization, Burt (1985) developed a simple method that local jurisdictions could use to calculate the cost of first births to teenagers *within their jurisdiction* within a given year or for a given year's birth cohort over 20 years. Many jurisdictions actually made these calculations and used them to lobby their legislative bodies for more resources to address the problem. One particularly telling example was a small rural jurisdiction in a conservative state, where it was very difficult to get any resources either for pregnancy prevention or to help teen mothers stay in school. After making the calculations for the 20-year projection, the jurisdiction realized that it was spending *more than $1 million in welfare benefits for each and every birth cohort,* without even knowing it and without helping anyone very much. The size of this inadvertent "investment" got the attention of local policy makers, and funding for more appropriate services followed.

If we are able to create some viable models for estimating the payoffs of adolescent vulnerability, and compare them to investments in youth (always assuming that we can make the connection between the investment and desirable outcomes), we will be in a position to use these figures to influence policy. We do not want to make this endeavor seem too complicated, but we do not want to make it seem too simple either. During the past decades, a body of literature has been building to indicate the complexities of youth behavior patterns and the inadequacy of single-problem approaches to understanding risk and vulnerability (Catalano et al., 1999). Those complexities multiply when we begin to think about outcomes and associated payoffs, but only by considering the complexities are we likely to get within shooting range of a reasonable estimate of payoffs.

The Approaches We Will Explore

We will try to develop a hybrid approach to assessing payoffs of investing in youth that avoids the disadvantages of some classic economics formulations of cost-benefit analysis. We want to be able to identify the payoffs of youth risk behavior to the public purse, but we also want to capture the broader context that includes personal or private costs and benefits. The reasons for these preferences will be detailed later in this paper. Furthermore, we will examine the payoffs of *patterns* of youth risk behavior, rather than of a single type of risk behavior. The reasons for this approach should be obvious from the results of the past decades of research on youth risk behaviors and evaluations of programs taking a single-focus versus a holistic approach to promoting positive youth outcomes.

Our approach involves modeling a conceptual framework containing three sets of transitional probabilities: (1) from antecedent risk factors to risk behavior patterns; (2) from risk behavior patterns to outcomes (pregnancy, addiction, suicide, jail, CEO of Fortune 500 company); (3) and from outcomes to payoffs (probability of using or contributing to public resources/well-being, private resources/well-being).

The Structure of This Paper

The remainder of this paper is structured to address the three components of our conceptual framework. The first component goes from risk/vulnerability factors to risky behavior; that is, it should be able to model the transitional probabilities that certain behaviors or patterns of behavior will emerge, given the existence of certain antecedent conditions. We treat this component very lightly, as these issues have been the focus of a great deal of research. In addition, the paper by Blum, McNeely, and Nonnemaker in this volume summarizes these issues in sufficient detail.

The second component goes from risk behaviors or patterns to outcomes, both positive and negative. We must determine the likelihood that any given behavior, repeated behavior, or pattern of behaviors will result in particular outcomes. Part of this task includes the important element of estimating co-occurrence or patterning of behaviors. This is essential because the synergies or interactions of certain behaviors in the presence of other behaviors may be more likely to produce costly consequences than if the focal behavior occurred in isolation. For instance, risky sexual behavior may lead to pregnancy, or to sexually transmitted diseases (STDs). Risky sexual behavior in combination with serious use of illegal drugs may add addiction, problems with a pregnancy, a child suffering the effects of fetal drug exposure, prison time for the mother, and a fractured family unit to the "simple" costs of pregnancy or treatment for STDs. Relatively little work of this type has been done to date, but some data sets exist that could be used to begin relevant analyses.

The third component is even more challenging, and less explored, than the second one. That is to translate outcomes of risk behavior patterns into payoffs. Our presentation here will be almost totally speculative. It will cover the probability of using and/or contributing to public resources in various arenas (education, health, mental health, criminal justice, social services, cash benefits, and so on, as well as taxes paid, contributions to community well-being, becoming an employer of others, and other fanciful conceptions). It also will cover the probability of incurring private costs (e.g., costs of health insurance, income foregone) and/or reaping private benefits (e.g., earnings, long life, benefits to children of stable families). It will attempt to present models projecting over a person's lifetime. It will attempt to meet various challenges such as "payoffs of adolescent risk behaviors to/for whom?" and "compared to what?" It will attempt to model ways to compare the cost of various investments that could be made in youth throughout their adolescence to their potential long-term effects on payoffs in adulthood. It will raise issues of who must make the decision to invest in adolescents versus who will incur the costs or reap the benefits of these investments in later years. It certainly will not succeed to everyone's (anyone's?) satisfaction, but it will be an interesting beginning.

This Paper Is Hypothetical—Data Will Come Later

Our task in this paper is to develop one or more frameworks for analyzing the payoffs of adolescent behavior and the outcomes that follow from it in adulthood. We are also to suggest the types of data we would need to gather if we want to estimate any of the models that we will suggest. We were not charged with actually *doing* any data analysis—just with thinking through and laying out what it would take to "do it right." Readers may have their own ideas for modifying the models we present, or their own sources of data for beginning the work of estimating all or part of our models. If we succeed in stimulating a new spurt of activity modeling payoffs of investing in adolescents, this paper will have done its job.

FROM VULNERABILITY FACTORS TO RISK BEHAVIORS

Past research has identified a number of vulnerability factors that increase the likelihood that youth will participate in health risk behaviors. It has shown that many of the same vulnerability factors predict a variety of health risks and related outcomes, such as substance use, delinquency, violence, adolescent pregnancy, and dropping out of school (Catalano et al., 1999). Over the course of the past decades, researchers also have sought to identify protective factors that help prevent youth from taking risks. Two recent analyses have moved to the forefront of the discussion on predictors of adolescent risk-taking behavior. Using data from the National Longitudinal Study of Adolescent Health (Add Health), both Resnick and colleagues (1997) and Blum and colleagues (2000) found that demographic variables (race/ethnicity, family income, and family structure) are only weakly related to adolescent risk-taking behaviors such as substance use, risky sexual activity, and violence. Additionally, Resnick, Blum, and others have found that processes such as family connectedness, school connectedness, and time spent in structured activity work to reduce the amount of risky behavior among youth.

Although the above research sheds light on predictors of risk-taking behaviors one at a time, it is not clear if the predictors hold when capturing the multidimensional nature of adolescent risk-taking behavior. Building on the seminal work of Jessor and Jessor (1977) on the co-occurrence of risk-taking behaviors, many researchers have documented links and patterns among various behaviors. These patterns of co-occurrence include aggression, substance use, and suicidal behavior (Garrison et al., 1993); substance use, sexual activity, and suicidal behavior (Burge et al., 1995); substance use and violence (Durkham et al., 1996); and substance use and sexual activity (Shrier et al., 1996). Jessor and colleagues (1977, 1991) speculated that youth risk taking comprises a single syndrome of problem behaviors, or as Elliot (1993) described it, a single health-compromising lifestyle.

Pursuing this direction of inquiry further, Zweig et al. (2001a) decided to model the reality of adolescent risk taking. We attempted to capture the multidimensional nature of youth risk taking using Add Health data and cluster analysis. We found that youth participate in both health-enhancing lifestyles (Elliot, 1993) and a variety of different health-compromising lifestyles that we have called health risk profiles. We examined sexual activity, general alcohol use, binge drinking, cigarette use, marijuana use, other illicit drug use, fighting, and suicide for female and male students in grades 9 through 12. Four distinct profiles were identified for females and four for males (Figures 4-1 and 4-2). The four risk profiles for females included: (1) a low-risk, sexually active group (having used contraception during both their first and most recent sexual experiences, if sexually active); (2) a low-risk group, with higher levels of fighting and of suicidal thoughts and behaviors; (3) a moderate-risk group, with higher levels of substance use and risky sexual behavior; and (4) a high-risk group across all risk behaviors. The four risk profiles for males included: (1) a low-risk group across all behaviors; (2) a moderate-risk group with higher levels of alcohol use, binge drinking, cigarette use, and risky sexual behavior; (3) a moderate-risk group with higher levels of marijuana use and of suicidal thoughts and behaviors; and (4) a high-risk group with low levels of suicidal thoughts and behaviors.

Once we identified adolescent health risk profiles, we too wanted to know about the vulnerability and protective factors related to each. Like our colleagues, we found that demographic factors such as age, race/ethnicity, and family income did not distinguish the profiles in meaningful ways (Zweig et al., 2001b). Also like our colleagues, we found that other processes predicted differences in profiles, and we have been able to make clearer distinctions about what factors predict particular lifestyles. Youth in low-risk profiles and profiles distinguished by substance use and sexual activity reported higher levels of individual psychosocial adjustment, family

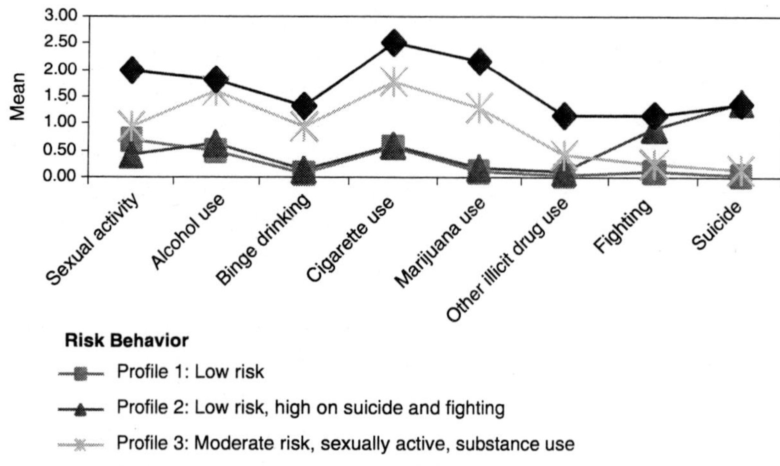

FIGURE 4-1 Profiles of risk—Females grades 9-12.
SOURCE: Zwieg, J. M., Lindberg, L. D., & McGinley, K. L. (2001). Used with permission of the *Journal of Youth and Adolescence.*

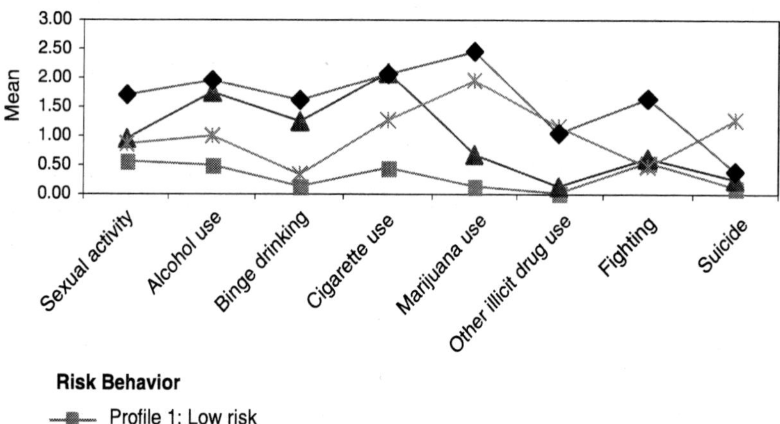

FIGURE 4-2 Profiles of risk—Males grades 9-12.
SOURCE: Zwieg, J. M., Lindberg, L. D., & McGinley, K. L. (2001). Used with permission of the *Journal of Youth and Adolescence.*

connectedness, and school connectedness than students in high-risk profiles and profiles distinguished by suicidal thoughts and behaviors.

The important message from our analysis is that teens in low-risk profiles and profiles distinguished by substance use and sexual activity are similar, and at relatively low risk—they consistently report lower levels of vulnerability factors and higher levels of protective factors than other teens. Some teens who have sex and use alcohol and tobacco have as few vulnerabilities and as many protective factors as teens who participate in little or no risk behavior. Teens in high-risk profiles and profiles distinguished by suicidal thoughts and behaviors are also similar—teens in both groups consistently report higher levels of vulnerability factors and lower levels of protective factors. Teens who are suicidal but do not report participating in any other risk behaviors are as vulnerable and unprotected as those who participate in all types of risk behaviors.

FROM HEALTH RISK PATTERNS TO OUTCOMES

Thus far we have discussed the evidence that youth participate in both health-enhancing and health-compromising lifestyles and that membership in groups based on these lifestyles can be predicted by vulnerability and protective factors operating in the lives of youth. Next we must establish the probability that these lifestyles will lead to particular outcomes and patterns of outcomes. To date, whenever we have thought about assessing the public burden of adolescent risk, it usually has been done with one risk behavior or one outcome in mind. Private payoffs largely have been ignored. But we know that youth participate in different lifestyles comprising various combinations of behaviors, some more risky than others. These health-compromising and health-enhancing lifestyles can lead to combinations of both negative and positive outcomes that can contribute to or help reduce the public burden or general social welfare outcomes of youth behavior. To understand the scope of outcomes youth may face as a result of their risk-taking behavior, we cannot examine one risk or one outcome at a time. Rather, we must keep their risk-taking patterns in mind, and attempt to link these to all possible related outcomes. By linking lifestyles to the many outcomes that may result, we will more realistically discuss adolescent risk taking, its outcomes, and its payoffs.

So, how do we link adolescent lifestyles to outcomes, and thence to their associated payoffs? First we need to know what information exists (in the form of results from previous analyses or actual data that lend themselves to the necessary analyses) that allows us to identify adolescent lifestyles and link these to possible outcomes associated with each. Then, once we establish relationships between lifestyles and outcomes, we can incorporate the known probabilities in our model estimating payoffs.

National data sets may provide some of the answers when it comes to linking lifestyles and outcomes, but no one data set has all the necessary information. Some data sets can only be assessed for shorter term outcomes, while others can be assessed for both shorter and longer term outcomes depending on the length of the longitudinal study. Furthermore, some data sets are much richer with respect to some outcomes than to others (e.g., economic behavior versus sexual behavior versus criminal or violent behavior). Therefore, we will almost certainly have to use more than one data set to understand the full range of outcomes. This necessity leads in turn to the need to resolve a number of methodological issues. For example, different measures have been used across studies to assess adolescent risk-taking behavior, making it more or less difficult to model adolescent health-compromising and health-enhancing lifestyles. The lifestyles identified in one data set may not be comparable to those identified in another data set.

In addition, when relying on older data sets to assess longer term outcomes, we must remember that the youth of interest were participating in risky behavior 20 years ago. The meaning of adolescent risk taking and its associated outcomes may have changed since then. More current data provide information about how risk behaviors have shifted over time. For example, recent trends in adolescent risk taking indicate decreases in some risk behaviors such as violence and sexual activity, and increases in others such as substance use (Boggess et al., 2000). Therefore, although we may be able to measure the same age groups, differences of cohort and time may make it difficult to compare results across data sets and tell a full story of the payoffs of adolescent risk (Baltes et al., 1977).

Data options that may be relevant to the current effort are discussed in the following paragraphs.

1. *National Longitudinal Study of Adolescent Health* (Add Health: http://www.cpc.unc.edu/addhealth)

Add Health was designed to examine adolescent physical, mental, emotional, and reproductive health. Add Health's first wave of data collection was completed in 1994-95. That year, 90,000 youth completed in-school surveys about their background, friends, school life, school work and activities, and general health status. Of these youth, 21,000 also participated in an in-home survey about family and peer relationships, school environment, health risk behaviors (including sexual activity, violence, and substance use), psychosocial adjustment, physical health, and perceptions of risk. Wave II was completed in 1996, a year after Wave I. Wave III is currently in the works and will be collected in 2001, with youth now young adults approximately between the ages of 18 and 24.

Add Health is an exceptional data set to identify lifestyles of youth risk taking, and indeed, we have already done this with Wave I data. Until Wave III is completed, however, little can be done to assess outcomes of these lifestyles given that Wave II was collected only one year after the first wave. The Wave III data are an excellent resource to help us understand the shorter term health-related outcomes of youth risk (such as teen pregnancy and STDs) and educational and work histories thus far. In addition, we may know about participants' financial situations, health insurance, and use of public programs. Less will be known about participants' criminal behavior and history, however, and we will also not know about the longer term outcomes of adolescent lifestyles given the length of the project thus far.

2. *National Survey of Adolescent Males* (NSAM: http://www.nichd.nih.gov)

NSAM was designed to assess male adolescent risk taking and reproductive health. To date, it includes three waves of data collection, with Wave I completed in 1989 when males were 15 to 19 years old. Wave II was collected in 1990-91 and Wave III was collected in 1995. A new second cohort of males ages 15 to 19 were also added at Wave III. Participants were asked about their background, educational history and aspirations, sexual activity, substance use, attitudes about contraception and gender roles, and knowledge about sexual activity, contraception, and AIDS.

Like Add Health, NSAM would be an appropriate data set to identify adolescent health-compromising and health-enhancing lifestyles, but also like Add Health, the participants were only followed through young adulthood, allowing assessment of only shorter term outcomes related to risk. In addition, use of social programs, violence, criminal behavior, employment, and suicide ideation are not identified as areas of focus for the study, so presumably we have less information on these issues.

3. *National Longitudinal Survey of Youth* (NLSY: http://www.bls.gov.nlsy)

The NLSY began in 1979 to examine labor force participation and related activities of youth. Approximately 13,000 youth ages 14 through 21 were surveyed at the time and have participated in a total of 17 waves of data collection. The last wave was in 1998 when participants were between 33 and 40 years old. Participants have been asked about their educational and employment histories, income and assets, use of public programs, child care, health conditions, substance use, sexual activity, marriage, and fertility. Since 1986, children of the women in the NLSY study have been surveyed as well. Six waves of data collection on children from birth to age 14 have been included. The children's surveys include assessments of cognitive, socioemotional, and physiological well-being. In addition, in 1997, a second cohort of 9,000 youth ages 12 to 16 began to be studied. Three waves of data collection have been completed to date.

Identifying health-compromising and health-enhancing lifestyles using the NLSY may be more difficult than using Add Health or NSAM. Although participants were asked about substance use and sexual activity, violence and suicidal behavior are not identified as study focuses. However, NLSY would be an exceptional data set to map outcomes to lifestyles because both shorter and longer term outcomes can be assessed. In addition, outcomes for children can be incorporated into models. Importantly, outcomes related to use of social programs, health, employment, and education all can be assessed. However, outcomes related to crime and delinquency may not be readily accessible.

4. *National Youth Survey* (NYS: http://www.icpsr.umich.edu)

The NYS was designed to assess both conventional and deviant youth behaviors. It includes multiple waves of data collection beginning in 1976, when approximately 2,000 youth were ages 9 to 18. The last wave of data that is available for public use at this time was collected in 1987, when participants were ages 20 to 29. Currently, an eleventh wave of data are being collected with participants between the ages of 34 to 43. Participants were asked about background information, friends and family, neighborhood issues, education, employment, psychosocial adjustment, delinquency, substance use, sexual activity, pregnancy and abortion, use of mental health services, and violence. Like Add Health and NSAM, NYS would be an appropriate data set to identify adolescent lifestyles. But unlike Add Health and NSAM, we could map both shorter and longer term outcomes related to adolescent lifestyles into young adulthood and middle adulthood. However, we assume that less information is available on use of public programs in this data set.

5. *Literature Search on Outcomes*

Another way to identify outcomes would be to review the literature linking individual risk behaviors with particular outcomes. A thorough review of the literature would help us assess the magnitude and consistency of the relationships between individual behaviors and outcomes; however, we would not be able to examine adolescent behaviors as different lifestyles with all of their associated outcomes. We could only generate probabilities of individual behaviors and outcomes that could then be used in models assessing the payoffs of adolescent risk. Although this would be one way to identify probabilities, it is less desirable than generating the probabilities from the actual data presented earlier and based on lifestyles.

Although a great deal of analysis is not available at this date that does the work of understanding how different health risk profiles link to different outcome sets, the foregoing should clarify that some resources are at hand to remedy this gap in the available literature. Most important, it appears to be possible with existing data sets to begin the work of mapping complex health risk profiles onto equally complex multidimensional outcome sets. This is a matter of identifying multidimensional probability distributions on both sides, rather than the much simpler task of estimating the separate probabilities that one type of risk behavior will lead to various different undesirable outcomes, taken one at a time. Nevertheless, the challenge appears to us to be one well worth taking on, and one for which we have a fair probability of moving the field several steps forward. However, we have yet another step to take, and that is to payoffs. The next section moves us in this direction.

FROM OUTCOMES TO PAYOFFS

It will be no small task to accomplish the mapping of outcomes onto risk profiles. But at least that task is conceptually clear and can be undertaken without needing to make major decisions as to its nature. Such clarity has not yet come to the next, and last, task we describe in this paper—that of moving from outcomes to payoffs.

We start by parsing the task into two subtasks, one of which itself will need to be divided further. The first subtask is to attach payoffs to the various sets of outcomes developed from the work described. The second subtask is to analyze the payoffs from various types of investment in youth. In describing this second subtask, we will adopt the simplifying assumption that there are two major approaches for programs directed toward youth that we want to assess: (1) "classic" prevention of unwanted behaviors; and (2) promoting positive youth development. The first approach is most similar to many programs in the past—prevention programs targeted toward the highest risk youth. These programs usually aim to prevent bad outcomes, intervene after youth behavior has already reached the "risky" level, and have relatively little focus on promoting good outcomes. The second approach incorporates the latest thinking about positive youth development, including the desire to help large segments of the most disadvantaged youth in this country to move toward healthy and productive adulthood, not just avoid negative outcomes. The different conceptions of programming for youth lend themselves to quite different approaches to modeling investments and payoffs, at least as a first take.

Attaching Payoffs to Individual Outcomes and Outcome Patterns

The first step we must take to develop this analysis for investing in youth is simply to model the payoffs[1] associated with a set of outcomes. To begin, we have borrowed from Cohen's (2000) work describing the costs and benefits of crime, and expanded it to include an array of payoffs particular to adolescents (Table 4-1). These payoffs are divided into domains, and the domains are further divided into payoff categories. The categories are not intended to be exhaustive, but rather to list some major payoffs associated with each domain.

Next we must specify who gets the payoffs associated with a particular domain or outcome. At this point, if we consulted the cost-benefit literature, which comes mainly from economics, we would be presented with two choices—"the public," meaning government, and "society," meaning people as private agents and markets as markets, but NOT government.

Because we began work on this paper thinking we were interested in

---

[1]We use the word "payoffs" to clarify that the distinction between a cost and a benefit is artificial: costs are simply values associated with negative outcomes and benefits are values associated with positive outcomes. A cost can be either a direct cost (such as Medicaid expenditures for drug-involved adolescents) or a benefit that does not occur (such as ill health among adolescents who were expected to be healthy). Similarly, a benefit can be either a direct benefit (earnings of adolescents helped to complete schooling) or a cost that does not occur (reduced unemployment or costs of crime)

TABLE 4-1 Payoffs Associated with the Outcomes of Adolescent Vulnerability

Domain	Payoff of:	Payoff to/for Whom?	Existing Estimates
Crime	Arrest/prosecution	Y/SPUB	Limited
	Detention	Y/SPUB	Yes
	Security	C/SPRI/SPUB	Yes
	Victimization	C	Yes
Education	Literacy	Y/C/SPUB/SPRI	Yes
	GED	Y/C/SPUB/SPRI	Yes
	High school graduation	Y/C/SPUB/SPRI	Yes
	College graduation	Y/C/SPUB/SPRI	Yes
	Productivity	Y/C/SPUB/SPRI	Limited
Employment	Productivity	Y/C/SPUB/SPRI	Limited
	Wages	Y/C/SPUB	Yes
	Taxes	Y/C/SPUB	Yes
	Unemployment	Y/C/SPUB	Yes
Family	AFDC	SPUB	Limited
	Child support	Y/C/SPUB/SPRI	Limited
	Stable families	Y/C	??
Health	Insurance	Y/SPRI	Yes
	Medicaid/SSI	SPUB	Limited
	Productivity	Y/C/SPUB/SPRI	Limited
	Mortality (YLL)	Y/C	Yes
	Healthy children	Y/C/SPUB/SPRI	Yes
	Lost Wages	Y/SPUB	Yes
Other (Externalities)	Resource choices "Social value" factor	Individual/public	Limited

NOTES: Y = Youth; C = Community; SPUB = Society/Public Sector; SPRI = Society/Private Individuals and Others. GED = General Education Development Tests; AFDC = Aid to Families with Dependent Children; SSI = Supplemental Security Income; YLL = Years of Life Lost.

"public burden," it is important at this point to explain why we are about to deviate from that intention. As noted, the public burden approach considers only payoffs to government; it does not capture values to individuals. If we were interested only in discussing payoffs from public investment in prevention programs, especially secondary and tertiary prevention, we would probably be content with a "public burden" approach. We would be most interested in public costs averted, which the approach would capture. We also would expect little from these programs by way of generating positive social welfare (e.g., more self-sufficient individuals, more viable communities and families), and thus would not be disappointed when the public burden approach failed to capture these benefits.

However, we also want to be able to model the payoffs of programs and activities based on a positive youth development approach. Such programs are more likely than prevention programs to serve a broader array of youth, to start younger and stay longer, and perhaps to take as their focus families, whole communities, neighborhoods, or schools. The activities they pursue with youth are different, in part, and their goals are less simple prevention and more promotion of individual and family competencies and well-being in adolescence and adulthood. They also often incorporate an interest in promoting community well-being. Many of the benefits of these approaches will not "register" at all in a public burden model of cost-benefit analysis. However, the main alternative approach in economics, the social welfare approach, is also inadequate for our purposes. It does not "register" public costs, and we are very interested in such costs.

Therefore we believe it is important to propose a hybrid approach, in which we name various potential beneficiaries of intervention and anticipate identifying the payoffs that each might expect from one or another type of intervention with youth. We propose to divide the expected payoff recipients into four groups, which we believe will provide the greatest clarity in examining the distribution of value throughout society (Table 4-1, column 3). These four groups are (1) youth themselves (Y), who might be affected directly by a program; (2) the immediate community (C) in which the youth reside, including their peers, families, and local institutions; and (3 and 4) the rest of society. Values accruing to "the rest of society" may be private (accruing to individuals) or public (accruing to governments) (SPRI and SPUB).

Table 4-1 reveals several points of interest. First, it is clear that in many domains, payoffs are anticipated across two, three, or all four of the groups. Second, the final column of Table 4-1 identifies whether a body of literature exists from which the payoffs associated with each of these events can be identified. It is clear that a body of literature already exists that can help us piece together the magnitude of each payoff. Third, it is clear that it may be easier to attach payoffs to a particular payer in some domains than in others. For example, health costs are categorized by payer, as this is relatively easy to do within this domain. It is rather harder to do so in the other domains, so the categories reflect the key areas where payoffs accrue (such as in the crime or education categories).

Finally, it is clear that a whole set of payoffs does not fall easily within any of these categories, but may fall into the "other" category. For instance, we may attach a positive social value to a flatter income distribution, or to having neighborhoods that function as viable communities. These can be represented in Table 4-1 as a "social value" function, whose actual value always will be a matter of opinion as opposed to fact. What the final column of Table 4-1 does suggest, however, is that enough knowledge exists to warrant attempts to model the payoffs of adolescent vulnerability, once we can establish sets of outcomes we want to "price."

To pursue our example of payoffs associated with a program designed to prevent criminal behavior in adolescents (Cohen, 2000), a list of negative payoffs might yield the following:

- Direct costs of program operation;
- Indirect costs of program operation (including the opportunity cost to society of not using the program's operating resources in their next best use);
- Foregone benefits to society due to reduced market efficiency as a result of collecting tax revenue for use in the program;
- Foregone benefit from bureaucratic "leakage" in administering these revenues;
- Foregone benefits to the program's participants in terms of opportunity costs in the present (costs of time spent in the program) and in the future; and
- Costs to public and private programs of services and benefits to which youth and their families gain access through program efforts.

The list of positive payoffs might include:

- Increased lifetime earnings;
- Increased taxes paid to government;

- Decreased costs associated with averted mortality and morbidity;
- Improved quality of life for youth themselves (including a more stable family or better outcomes for children of adolescents);
- Improved quality of life for community (including nonlinear effects of improved youth behavior, such as "tipping" the neighborhood in the good direction);
- Decreased public costs for services and benefits not needed by youth, their families, and their communities;
- Averted criminal justice costs, including costs associated with victimization, arrest, and incarceration; and
- Reduced market inefficiency due to taxes not being collected to provide revenues for transfer programs.

Sources of Information About Program Impact

Having addressed some of the major issues of what payoffs to include, and for whom, we still face the formidable problem of where to get reliable and generalizable information about the effects of interventions. At the beginning of this section, we described the first task of a payoff analysis as documenting the payoffs of outcomes in the present world, presumably in the absence of major interventions of the type we would like to contemplate. But obtaining that information is only half the battle. We also need information about the ability of programs to change the probabilities that certain outcomes will happen—reducing negative outcomes and their associated costs, and/or increasing positive outcomes and their associated benefits. This information is essential if we are to model the deviations from "normal" that are expected to result from various interventions.

However, if the cost-benefit literature is fraught with difficulties, the evaluation literature is equally unreliable. Conducting good evaluations is expensive in comparison to program costs, so relatively few are done. This means that any evaluation results that do exist are likely to concern exemplary or even special demonstration programs, rather than any "average" approach to intervening with youth. Thus, any documented program effects may depend on aspects of the program that *cannot* readily be replicated elsewhere. In addition, when model programs are "adapted" into general use, they are nearly always diluted, sometimes beyond recognition. This dilution nearly always relates to the cost of the original program (usually high) and the unwillingness or inability of the adapting jurisdictions or organizations to commit the same amount of resources to the program.

(That is, they want the name, but not the game.) As a consequence, it is not so surprising that the second and subsequent generations of model programs do not produce the same results. Therefore we face major issues related to both the *generalizability of evaluation results* and the *effects of going to scale.*

Nevertheless, we should be able to pose the hypothetical case that IF a community implemented a program of known effects with reasonable fidelity to the original (including what it cost), we could expect it to produce the results documented by the evaluation. In addition, we could easily calculate the benefits to be expected from a reduction of X percent in the proportion of youth exhibiting a particularly hazardous health risk profile, or an increase of Y percent in the proportion exhibiting profiles of very low risk. For the purpose of articulating the probable benefits of intervention, calculations of this type might be enough to win an argument about how important it is to invest in youth.

Challenges and Precautions

Although we can frame a conceptual approach to cost-benefit analysis related to programming for youth, many practical obstacles interpose themselves between conception and execution.

Uncertainties

Several types of uncertainty present challenges to producing an accurate cost-benefit analysis. The first of these concerns *uncertainty about the actual occurrence of events in the future.* Because we are proposing to estimate payoffs over the lifetimes of youth who may be affected by interventions, this type of uncertainty will be very significant. It is, indeed, the reason why we propose the analyses that take up the middle section of this paper—those estimating the probability of certain outcomes, given certain behaviors. We expect these estimates to be a challenge in themselves, but if researchers succeed in making them, and in describing the timeframes during which they may be likely to occur, the work will have been done to meet this type of uncertainty within the cost-benefit framework.

The second type of uncertainty concerns the "half-life" of program effects. We know that the effects of program participation do not last forever. We suspect, and there is evidence to support this suspicion, that shorter interventions have shorter half-lives, and that major commitments to the lives of youth over time have more lasting effects. Also of interest is evidence that interventions based on positive youth development principles produce *increasingly positive* payoffs over time (that is, they set up "virtuous cycles"). The literature on *the longevity and direction of program effects* will need to be examined to see how long we may expect program efforts to affect outcomes, and the temporal patterning of effects if they are not linear (e.g., most early on, or most later on, interaction effects of program type or duration with effect type or duration).

The final type of uncertainty concerns *the appropriate discount rate* to use with current expenditures as they relate to benefits that will accrue in the future. This uncertainty concerns the value of money over time, which fluctuates with economic conditions and some government actions. Most analyses adopt some compromise "reasonable" rate, but the rate to use is always a judgment call, and yields more uncertain results the further into the future (and hence the further into uncertainty) a projection goes. This uncertainty also can be addressed by making estimates with high, low, and moderate rate assumptions and producing upper and lower bound estimates of payoffs as well as a middle-of-the-road result.

Intangibles

"Intangibles" are those things about which we all care passionately but on which we cannot put a price. "Public burden" analyses omit these payoffs entirely, while "social welfare" analyses struggle with how to place value on valuable but priceless things. These intangible costs or benefits are nontrivial, and thus must be addressed in some fashion. For example, Miller et al. (1996) note that the tangible costs associated with a single rape are about the same as those associated with a single motor vehicle theft. But once intangible costs such as pain and suffering are included, the costs associated with the rape are estimated to be more than 20 times that of the vehicle theft. Not surprisingly, substantial controversy surrounds the most appropriate method of measuring such intangible costs (see Roman et al., 1998).

Criteria for Decision Making

Even supposing that we can develop actual monetarized estimates for the outcomes of interventions to help youth, the question still remains of whether those investments are "worth it." Even more challenging may be choices that might have to be made between investing in one rather than another approach, assuming that both "work" to some extent. Suppose one had a classic prevention approach that was closely targeted on the worst youth, did not do anything for most youth, and succeeded in preventing several of those "worst youth" from fulfilling the worst, most costly, expectations for the outcomes of their behavior. And suppose another program, taking a positive youth development approach with all the youth in a particular neighborhood, succeeded in helping most of them graduate from high school, go on to college or into the labor market, and lead productive lives. One program averts a great cost associated with a few individuals; the other program promotes reasonable benefits for many individuals and their families and neighborhoods. Suppose the actual interventions require about the same level of investment and you only have enough resources for one of them. Which one do you choose? Obviously there is a correct answer to this from a monetarized point of view, but almost certainly the decision would not be made strictly on that basis.

Payoff Elements Critical to the Different Intervention Approaches

A cost-benefit analysis of an intervention program is obliged, at base, to use the program's model of its intentions as a blueprint for assessing whether achievements are worth the investment. If a program is trying to prevent drug abuse, it must be evaluated by the amount of drug use it has prevented, the costs of preventing it, and the benefits accruing from that prevention. If a program is trying to help inner-city children acquire an entrepreneurial spirit leading to initiating successful business endeavors, then a cost-benefit analysis must focus on those particular outcomes, their value, and the investments necessary to produce them.

Because the different approaches to intervening with at-risk youth have very different goals, it follows that a cost-benefit analysis assessing their impact will need to measure quite different outcomes. For the two generic types of intervention programs for youth, prevention and youth development, Table 4-2 gives a rough sense of the categories it will probably be important to value (identify costs or benefits for) and the entities to whom/which those values will accrue (youth, communities, and the public and private society sectors).

TABLE 4-2 Importance of Elements to "Classic" Prevention and Youth Development Models

Payoff Category		Prevention Model				Youth Development Model			
		Y	C	SPUB	SPRI	Y	C	SPUB	SPRI
Costs of the Intervention				H	H			H	H
Crime	Arrest/prosecution	H		H		H		H	
	Detention	H		H		H		H	
	Security			H	H			H	H
	Victimization		H				H		
Education	Literacy					H	H		
	GED					H	H		
	High school graduation					H	H		
	College graduation					H	H		H
	Productivity					H	H		H
Employment	Productivity					H	H		H

	Wages				H			
	Taxes		H				H	
	Unemployment	H	H		H	H	H	
Family/ Community	Supportive Communities					H		
	Child support				H			H
	Stable families				H	H		
	Means-tested benefits		H				H	
Health	Insurance			H			H	H
	Medicaid/SSI		H				H	
	Productivity			H	H	H		H
	Mortality (YLL)	H			H	H		
	Healthy children					H		H
	Lost wages	H			H			
Other	"Social welfare"					H		H

NOTES: Y = Youth; C = Community; SPUB = Society/Public Sector; SPRI = Society/Private Individuals and Others. H = important element for this model. GED = General Education Development Tests; SSI = Supplemental Security Income; YLL = Years of Life Lost.

HYPOTHETICAL MODELS

Most readers would probably benefit from some examples related to the foregoing discussion, preferably accompanied by visual aids. A very stylized "full model" is presented in Figure 4-3. The full model is then broken down into sections to indicate the beginnings of its complexity.

Figure 4-3, then, shows a relatively full model capable of "covering" traditional prevention programs and positive youth development programs, as well as many things in between and beyond. It starts with the typical antecedents of youth risk behavior, well known to researchers in the field. These antecedents are expected to influence the health risk profile that a youth reports (path A), and also to have direct effects on negative outcomes in adolescence and adulthood (path B). The health risk profile of a particular adolescent is expected to affect that adolescent's patterns of negative outcomes (path C) and positive outcomes (path D). In addition, this model treats resiliency factors as exogenous, and as moderators of the effects of health risk profiles on negative and positive outcomes (paths E). Finally, outcomes are associated with payoffs.

To illustrate the differential expectations of different health risk profiles on negative and positive outcomes in adolescence and adulthood, we selected several profiles from those illustrated in Figures 4-1 and 4-2. The first of these is a profile fitting both boys and girls who are sexually active but who use protection during sex and who use substances (alcohol, tobacco, and marijuana) at moderate levels. The youth exhibiting this profile are shown at the left of Figure 4-4 (modeling path C, from behaviors to negative outcomes) and Figure 4-5 (modeling path D, from behaviors to positive outcomes). The second profile, shown to the right in Figures 4-4 and 4-5, is for girls only who report high levels of suicidal ideation and attempts and also elevated levels of fighting with peers and siblings in various settings.

Without attempting to be empirically accurate but basing our judgments on a fairly extensive knowledge of the risk-to-outcome literature, we have drawn these figures to show the probabilities of various outcomes *as patterns, in response to the different patterns represented by the profiles.* Several points are important to make about these sets of probabilities. First, they are quite different for the different profiles. The profile to the left is expected to produce its greatest negative outcomes in the areas of cigarette addiction, and secondarily in abuse of or addiction to alcohol and other drugs and their associated morbidities. The paths to injury (from drunk

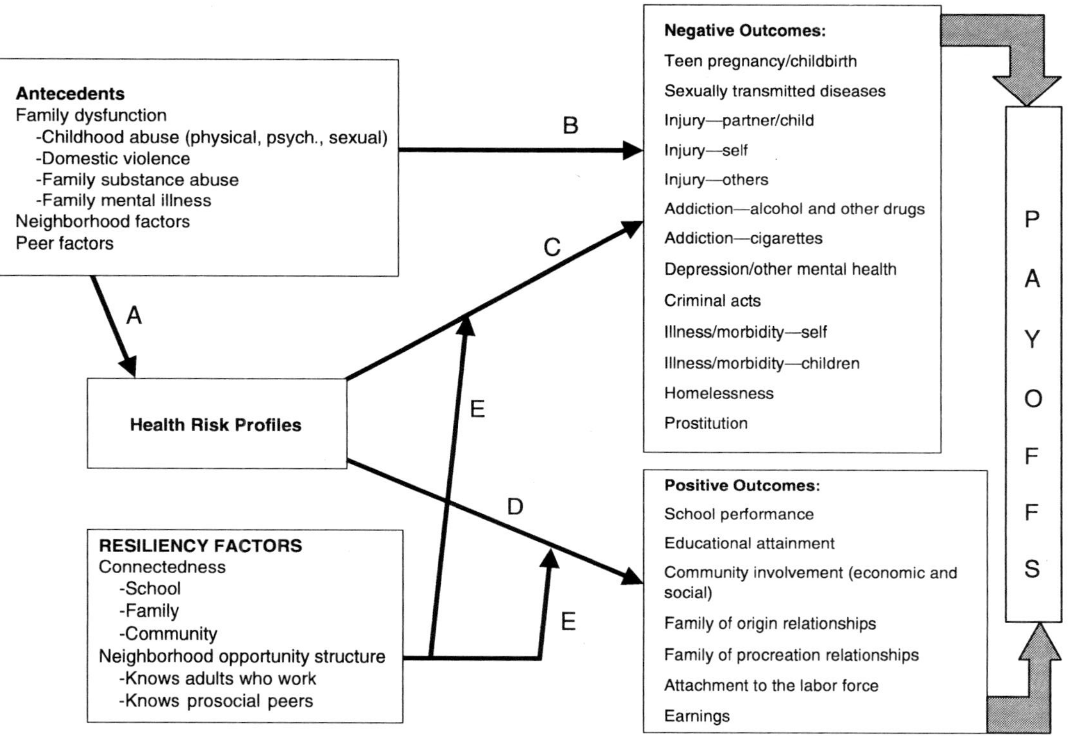

FIGURE 4-3 Modeling antecedents, behaviors, and outcomes.

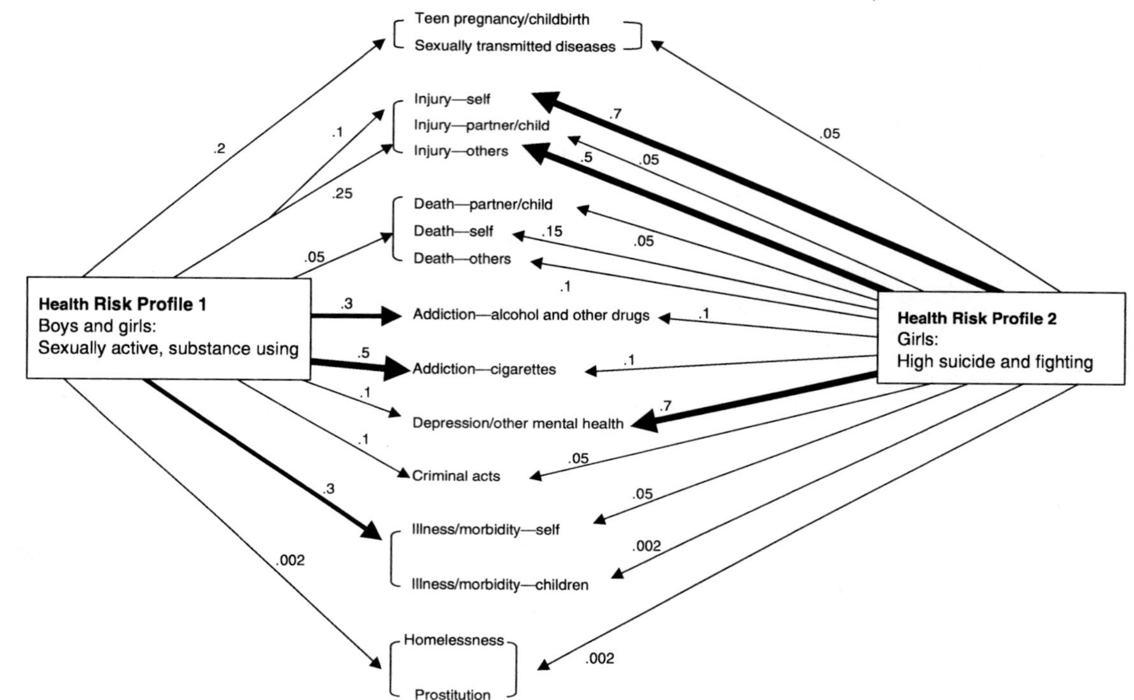

FIGURE 4-4 Modeling behaviors to negative outcomes, focusing on health risk effects and omitting effects of resiliency factors.

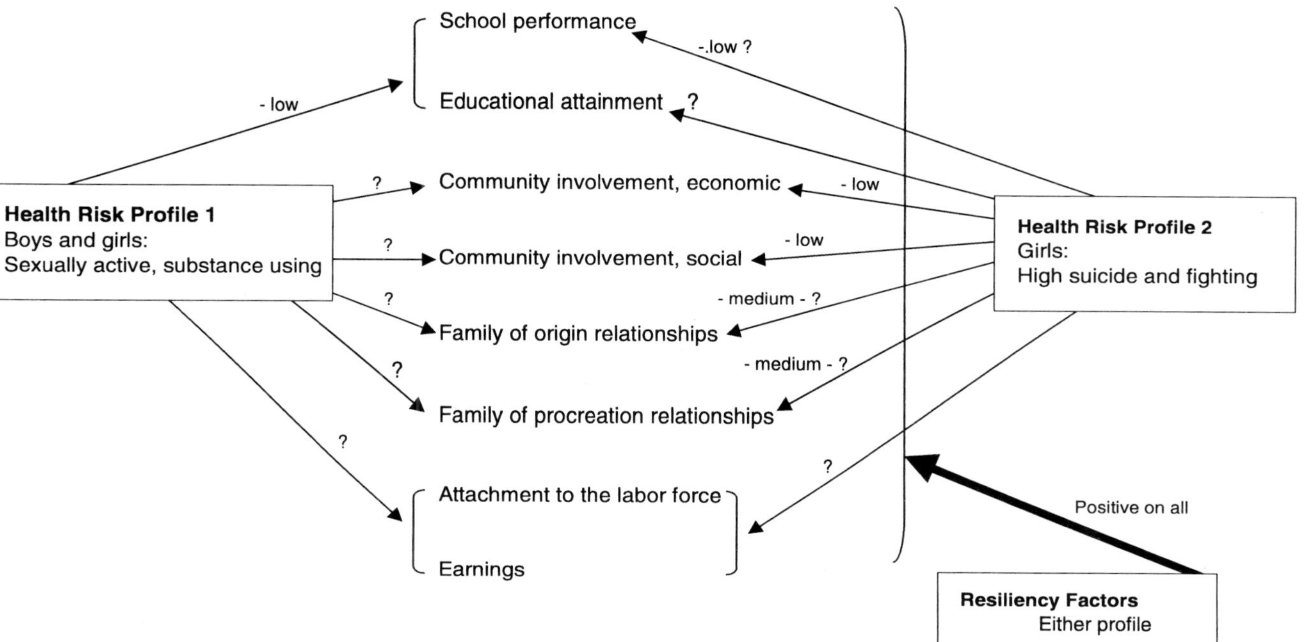

FIGURE 4-5 Modeling behaviors to positive outcomes, showing direct effects of resiliency factors.

driving, at the least) and pregnancy/STDs are also somewhat elevated. Interesting to us, as we tried to attach probabilities to Figure 4-5 for positive outcomes, is the relative lack of research documenting these, and we were forced to insert many question marks. The only fairly certain association is a negative one for school performance and educational attainment.

With respect to the second profile illustrated in Figures 4-4 and 4-5, the strongest associations are for physical injury to self or others, with an equally strong expectation of current and continuing mental health problems. Associations of this profile with positive outcomes were fairly speculative, but we mostly expected them to be negative (compared to youth with low-risk profiles). We expected that this profile could experience a fair degree of lowered outcomes in the area of family relationships, and also might be somewhat lower on community involvement.

We hope these profiles convey that behaviors occurring together in patterns may be expected to interact with each other to produce even more, or even less, of an outcome than would have occurred if one behavior occurred in isolation, as well as some outcomes that would not have occurred at all without both behaviors being present (e.g., babies born with fetal alcohol syndrome or crack addiction, in the case of the first profile). We did not include youth with the very highest risk profiles in these figures, basically because we could not fit in all of the very thick arrows we would have needed. However, we do expect that both boys and girls in these very high risk groups would exhibit very elevated levels of most of the negative outcomes and depressed levels of most of the positive outcomes.

The important thing to note is that we are going from one *pattern* (for behaviors) to another *pattern* (for outcomes), rather than from single behaviors to single outcomes. With respect to the associations of health risk profiles with negative outcomes, space and layout on the page did not let us show in Figure 4-4 the moderating effects of resiliency factors (paths E in Figure 4-3), because we would have had to draw arrows from resiliency factors to every arrow in the figure. Nor did we show the direct effects of antecedents (path B in Figure 4-3). Many more complexities would have been introduced had we done so, such as the possibility that sexual activity and substance use might escalate to prostitution and homelessness in the presence of physical or sexual abuse in the home environment, or that strong attachments to adults with pro-social values might provide the motivation to avoid pregnancy and substance abuse. Figure 4-5 does show the moderating effects of resiliency factors for positive outcomes because we had enough room on the page to do so.

Next we examine the types of payoffs that are most likely to be associated with particular outcomes (the final arrows in Figure 4-3). Table 4-3 shows the various positive and negative outcomes of our model as rows, and the various domains in which we can expect payoffs to occur as columns. Expectations for the intensity and direction of payoffs are indicated by plus and minus signs. Cells with a single minus sign indicate that we expect the outcome to produce net negative payoffs for that domain (e.g., pregnancy/teen childbearing/STDs in relation to family/community outcomes). Cells with a double minus sign indicate an expectation of strong negative payoffs. Conversely, cells with one or two plus signs indicate an expectation of positive payoffs. Cells without any sign indicate that we have no particular reason to expect unusual payoffs in that domain.

Needless to say, Table 4-3 is vastly oversimplified. It is probably no exaggeration to say that at least 10,000 decisions would need to be made before we could attach real payoffs to real outcomes. First we would need to specify all the elements of each outcome, on the basis of at least some justifying evidence. Second, we would have to specify all of the different types of crime, health, education, and other payoff types and subtypes. Third, we would have to attach a value to each, again on the basis of some evidence. Fourth, we would have to determine the probability that some entity would actually incur the payoffs, given that the outcome pattern happened. This sounds seriously intimidating, but at some level it is certainly possible.

Putting the Model Together with Interventions

The last thing to depict in this paper is the various paths that would have to be estimated to test the payoffs of different models of intervention with youth. We started this paper considering what we would need to do to show that investing in youth has important benefits for society. Figure 4-6 provides a schematic diagram of every component in our model; basically, this is what we would have to estimate to achieve the demonstration we seek.

Embedded in Figure 4-6 are two hypothetical "designs" for estimating payoffs. We spoke earlier of the traditional prevention approach and of the positive youth development approach, and specified in Table 4-2 how we expected payoffs to be distributed among the various recipients—youth, their community, the public sector, and the rest of society. One design, for an efficient (that is, an "indicated") prevention model, is shown by the

TABLE 4-3 Relationship of Outcomes to Payoff Domains

Outcome	Payoff Domain					
	Crime	Education	Employment	Family/ Community	Health	Other (Social Welfare)
Negative Outcomes						
Pregnancy/Teen Childbearing/STDs		— —	—	—	— —	—
Injury/Death		—	—	—	— —	—
Other Morbidity		—	—	—	—	
Addiction-AOD	—	—	—		— —	—
Addiction-Cigarettes					— —	
Mental Health	—	—	—	—	—	

Crime	— —					
Homelessness/ Prostitution, etc.	—			—	—	—
Positive Outcomes						
School Performance/ School Attainment	+	+ +	+ +	+		
Community Involvement	+		+	+ +		+
Family Relationships	+	+	+	+		+
Attachment to Labor Force/Earnings	+		+	+		+

NOTES: — = Negative payoffs/costs within a particular domain; + = Positive payoffs/benefits within a particular domain. Two signs (for example —) indicate a stronger relationship than a single sign. STDs = Sexually Transmitted Diseases; AOD = Alcohol and Other Drugs.

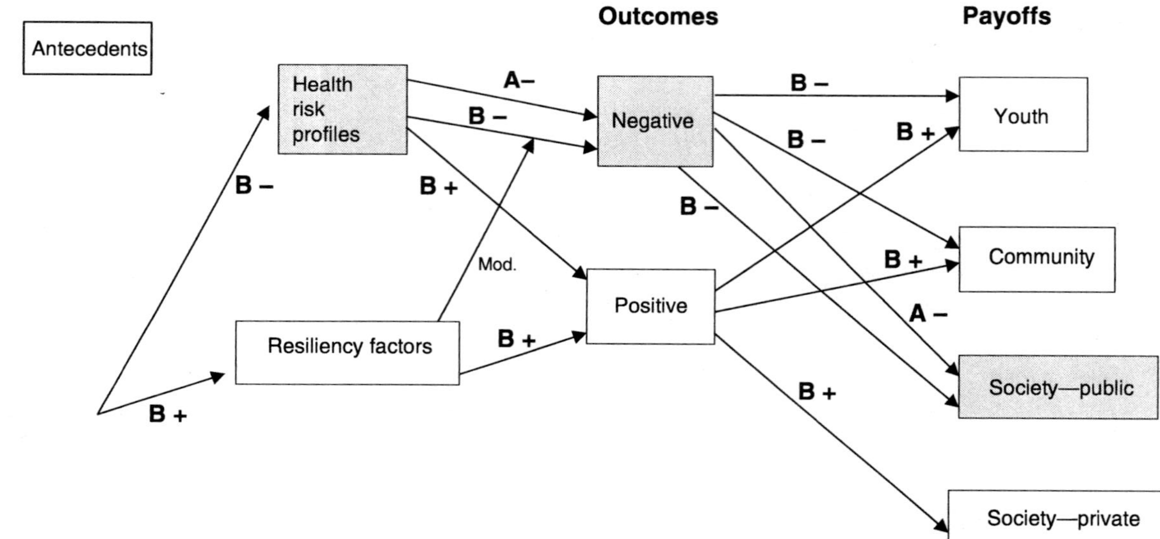

FIGURE 4-6 Alternative models of intervention and their implications for calculating payoffs.
NOTES: A = Point of intervention and payoff goals of typical "prevention" (tertiary attention/indicated intervention) program—reduce association between health risk profiles and negative outcomes, and reduce associated public costs. (Gray shaded boxes and the paths between.)
B = Points of intervention and payoff goals of youth development approach—increase resiliency factors, reduce less healthy risk profiles, increase positive as well as reduce negative outcomes, and reduce negative and increase positive payoffs for youth themselves, their communities, and the rest of society, as well as reducing public costs.

shaded boxes in Figure 4-6 and the two paths between them (labeled A). The direction of effect is shown by the signs, indicating that this prevention model tries to reduce the association between health risk profiles and negative outcomes, and thereby reduce the public costs associated with the negative outcomes. To see whether this approach "pays off," one would add up all the costs of the intervention itself, and weigh these against the net value of the payoffs to the various sectors that could benefit or be harmed by the outcomes.

The second design embedded in Figure 4-6, depicting a positive youth development approach, includes the same two pathways as for the indicated prevention approach, but also encompasses many other pathways and payoff recipients. Typical efforts of these programs start early and try to affect resiliency factors, behaviors, attitudes, relationships, and competencies leading to positive outcomes as well as reducing negative ones. The paths labeled "B" symbolize the goals of these programs—to increase payoffs for youth, communities, and the rest of society through creation of more positive outcomes, as well as to reduce public costs by reducing negative outcomes. In theory, to see whether this approach pays off, we follow the same tactics as we did for the indicated program. But obviously we have much more to identify, estimate, and calculate to achieve a full accounting of the payoffs of the second approach. The motivation to do so is that the payoffs potentially include much that is positive for communities and for society as a whole.

IMPLICATIONS—"WHERE TO NEXT?"

The "task" of justifying investment in youth, now that it is all laid out, seems quite enormous. But it also seems exciting, at least to the authors. Even thinking through what it would take, as skeletally as we have done it here, prompted many new thoughts and forced us to reconsider some ways we had thought about these issues before.

It is important to realize that although we have developed the model in a mostly linear fashion, it does not have to be researched that way. Researchers can take some of the newer pieces and work on them simultaneously. Thus we can be using existing databases to develop increasingly sophisticated analyses of associations between patterns of behavior and patterns of outcomes, at the same time that we are assembling existing literature to document the costs of various outcomes to different sectors and the probability that various outcomes will indeed lead to those costs. And we can think about and try to collect new data that we will need to turn these models into reality.

In addition, we can be doing more thinking about how to model the payoffs from different types of policy action. In the models presented here, we considered only "programs" involving fairly intensive face-to-face interactions among youth and others, including program staff, teachers, families, and others. We did not pay any attention to government actions such as pricing policies (raising the tax on cigarettes or alcohol, for example, as a deterrent to use). Nor did we consider the effects that changes in eligibility for benefit programs, such as the change from Aid to Families with Dependent Children (AFDC) to Temporary Assistance for Needy Families (TANF), might have on teen decision making about sexual behavior. Nor did we examine proposed "single bullet" solutions to certain problems such as "testing" (students, teachers, or both), "vouchers," or reducing school class size. In part, we have not done so because we believe the findings of decades that making a difference for at-risk youth means major investments in fairly complicated, intensive, enduring interventions. We don't think there are "single bullets." We also think it is quite difficult to take a very complex policy change such as federal welfare reform and attempt to articulate its effects on a single behavioral domain of a small part of its target population. Also, many such policies have a single focus (e.g., reduce teen smoking). Although this is an important goal, it is not likely to change the lives of the youth who most need help, and we chose to concentrate on programs with a chance of doing that. But others may choose to model the payoffs of these types of policy changes, and such modeling efforts are sure to advance the entire enterprise of estimating payoffs, which can only be good.

REFERENCES

Baltes, P. B., Reese, H. W., & Nesselroade, J. R. (1977). *Life-span developmental psychology: Introduction to research methods.* Hillsdale, NJ: Lawrence Erlbaum Associates.

Blum, R. W., Beuhring, T., Shew, M. L., Bearinger, L. H., Sieving, R. E., & Resnick, M. D. (2000). The effects of race/ethnicity, income, and family structure on adolescent risk behaviors. *American Journal of Public Health, 90*(12), 1879-1884.

Boggess, S., Lindberg, L. D., & Porter, L. (2000). Changes in risk-taking among high school students, 1991-1997: Evidence from the Youth Risk Behavior Surveys. In *Trends in well-being of America's children and youth 1999* (pp. 475-488). Washington, DC: Department of Health and Human Services.

Burge, V., Felts, M., Chenier, T., & Parillo, A. V. (1995). Drug use, sexual activity, and suicidal behavior in U.S. high school students. *Journal of School Health, 65*(6), 222-227.

Burt, M. R. (1985). *Teenage pregnancy: How much does it cost?* Washington, DC: Center for Policy Options.

Burt, M. R. (1986). Estimating the public costs of teenage childbearing. *Family Planning Perspectives, 18*(5), 221-226.

Burt, M. R., & Levy, F. (1987). Estimates of public costs for teenage childbearing: A review of recent studies and estimates of 1985 public costs. In S. L. Hofferth and C. Hayes (Eds.), *Risking the future: Adolescent sexuality, pregnancy and childbearing, Vol. II* (pp. 264-294). Committee on Child Development Research and Public Policy, Commission on Behavioral and Social Sciences and Education. Washington, DC: National Academy Press.

Catalano, R. F., Berglund, M. L., Ryan, J. A. M., Lonczak, H. S., & Hawkins, J. D. (1999). *Positive youth development in the United States: Research findings on evaluations of positive youth development programs.* Seattle, WA: Social Development Research Group.

Cohen, M. A. (1998). The monetary value of saving a high risk youth. *Journal of Quantitative Criminology, 14*(1), 5-33.

Cohen, M. A. (2000). Measuring the costs and benefits of crime and justice. In *Measurement and analysis of crime and justice, Volume 4: Criminal justice 2000.* NCJ 182410. Washington, DC: National Institute of Justice.

Durkham, C. P., Byrd, R. S., Auinger, P., & Weitzman, M. (1996). Illicit substance use, gender, and the risk of violent behavior among adolescents. *Archives of Pediatric and Adolescent Medicine, 150,* 797-801.

Elliot, D. S. (1993). Health-enhancing and health-compromising lifestyles. In S. G. Millstein, A. C. Petersen, & E. O. Nightingale (Eds.), *Promoting the health of adolescents: New directions for the twenty-first century* (pp. 112-145). New York, NY: Oxford University Press.

Garrison, C. Z., McKeown, R. E., Valois, R. F., & Vincent, M. L. (1993). Aggression, substance use, and suicidal behaviors in high school students. *American Journal of Public Health, 83*(2), 179-184.

Jessor, R. (1991). Risk behaviors in adolescence: A psychosocial framework for understanding and action. *Journal of Adolescent Health, 12,* 597-605.

Jessor, R., & Jessor. S. (1977). *Problem behavior and psychological development: A longitudinal study of youth.* San Diego, CA: Academic Press.

Miller, T. R., Cohen, M. A., & Wiersema, B. (1996). *Victim costs and consequences: A new look?* Washington, DC: Department of Justice, Office of Justice Programs, National Institute of Justice.

Millstein, S. G., Ozer, E. J., Ozer, E. M., Brindis, C. D., Knopf, D. K., & Irwin, C. E., Jr. (2000). *Research priorities in adolescent health: An analysis and synthesis of research recommendations, executive summary.* San Francisco: University of California, National Adolescent Health Information Center.

Resnick, M. D., Bearman, P. S., Blum, R. W., Bauman, K. E., Harris, K. M., Jones, J., Tabor, J., Beuhring, T., Sieving, R. E., Shew, M., Ireland, M., Bearinger, L. H., & Udry, J. R. (1997). Protecting adolescents from harm: Findings from the National Longitudinal Study of Adolescent Health. *Journal of the American Medical Association, 278*(10), 823-833.

Roman, J. Woodard, J., Harrell, A., & Riggs, S. (1998). *A methodology for measuring costs and benefits of court-based drug intervention programs using findings from experimental and quasi-experimental evaluations.* Washington, DC: Urban Institute.

Shrier, L. A., Emans, S. J., Woods, E. R., & DuRant, R. H. (1996). The association of sexual risk behaviors and problem drug behaviors in high school students. *Journal of Adolescent Health, 20,* 377-383.

Zweig, J. M., Lindberg, L. D., & McGinley, K. L. (2001). Adolescent health risk profiles: The co-occurrence of health risks among females and males. *Journal of Youth and Adolescence, 30*(6).

Zweig, J. M., Phillips, S. D., & Lindberg, L. D. (2001). *Predicting adolescent profiles of risk: Looking beyond demographics.* Washington, DC: Urban Institute. Paper prepared for the Department of Health and Human Services, Office of the Assistant Secretary for Planning and Evaluation.

5
Adolescent Vulnerability: Measurement and Priority Setting

Baruch Fischhoff and Henry Willis

INTRODUCTION

Adolescents face many threats to their health, safety, and well-being. Some are shared by their society as a whole (e.g., war, many diseases, crime). Others are unique to, or at least accentuated by, teens' transitions to arenas beyond the control of their guardians. Many adults devote much of their lives to reducing these vulnerabilities. There are school, community, and religious programs. There are medical screening, treatment, and educational efforts. There are lectures, remonstrations, and rescues by parents. There are special laws governing adolescent driving and status offenses. There are summits and conferences, some with teen representation, some without.

Teens often are described as living in a fog of exaggerated personal invulnerability (Millstein and Halpern-Felsher, this volume; Quadrel et al., 1993). However, both the scientific evidence and direct discussion show teens as having many legitimate concerns on their minds (Blum et al., this volume; Fischhoff et al., 1998, 2000). They wonder if and how they're going to get through this stage of their lives, with the world that they hope for reasonably intact. Chronic diseases are one part of that burden, especially when they induce moments of legitimate panic, like diabetes or asthma. Violence is another part, especially when teens feel as though they never know which minor incident (or sideways glance) is going to spin out of control. Fear about the continuity of the larger world is yet another part of the burden. It might weigh especially hard on teens attuned to signs of eroding faith in government, assaults on the natural world (and on animals, with which many young people feel a special affinity), turmoil in racial relations, or growing income inequality. Even with the recent economic boom for some, many teens must worry about having a decent career (not to mention a meaningful one).

These external concerns notwithstanding, teens obviously do not always act in ways that serve their own best interests, even in terms of the goals they set for themselves (which need not correspond to the goals that adults set for them). Worrying about life in general is not incompatible, with teens sometimes underestimating the risks posed by particular behaviors (e.g., unsafe sex, drinking and driving). Nor need teens' critical decisions be driven entirely by calm deliberation. Of course, adults, too, often have exaggerated feelings of control over life events and, occasionally, let emotion carry them away (Loewenstein, 1996; Weinstein, 1987). However, they may face a lower rate of fateful decisions than do young people, who are trying to set up their lives—including how they will deal with work, drugs, driving, drinking, and intimacy, among other things. Thus, teens themselves create risks that compound those that the world imposes on them.

THE NEED FOR INDICATORS

To deal effectively with these vulnerabilities, teens and adults need to know how big the threats are and how much can be done about them. That means knowing how big the *overall burden* of adolescent vulnerability is, in order to decide what personal and societal resources to devote to threats to adolescents (relative to other priorities). It means knowing the *relative size* of specific threats, and of the expected costs and benefits of opportunities for risk reduction, in order to identify the "best buys" in risk reduction. Where these questions cannot be answered confidently, better research is needed, for each link in the analytical chain. Systematic uncertainty reduction is the goal of research focused on patterns of problem behavior and predisposing conditions, creating either vulnerability or resilience (Blum et al., this volume; Jessor et al., 1991).

Where even the best buys are not very attractive, then social investments (including research) are needed to make better options available for youth. The shift from problem-focused interventions to positive youth development ones is a response to feelings of fundamental inadequacy in what we offer young people (Burt et al., this volume). A sweeping change in policy requires a comprehensive look at the evidence, expressed in some common and relevant terms. Realizing this, both national and international bodies have called for routine reporting of comparable statistics on critical indicators of youth welfare (e.g., Department of Health and Human Services, 2000; Federal Interagency Forum on Child and Family Statistics, 1997; United Nations, 1989). Suitably chosen indicators provide targets for social action and allow tracking of changes over time.

Identifying the critical indicators is also a necessary condition for communications focused on the facts the teens, adults, and policy makers most need to know (Fischhoff, 2000; Millstein and Halpern-Felsher, this volume). Without such analysis, people may be denied guidance for effective action. They may have their time and trust wasted by streams of irrelevant communications. They may be faulted for failing to know facts that were hardly worth knowing, yet found their way onto someone's improvised test of lay understanding. The resulting disrespect undermines respect for citizens and contributes to their disenfranchisement. It perpetuates a vicious circle, leading citizens to mistrust these dismissive experts, who fail to provide viable solutions or even needed information.

However, even the best data alone do not set priorities among threats to adolescents (or the natural environment or economic opportunity or anything else). Those priorities require value judgments regarding the relative importance of different outcomes. For example, Burt et al. (this volume) raise a not-so-hypothetical choice between two competing programs. One, focused on the most serious problem behaviors, could prevent "several of those 'worst youth' from fulfilling the worst, most costly, expectations for the outcomes of their behavior." The other, focused on positive youth development, could prevent many less challenged youth from failing to fulfill their potential ("graduate from high school, go on to college or into the labor market, and lead productive lives").

In a world of finite resources, such choices are inevitable. They face not only agencies with limited budgets, but also parents with limited time, energy, and interpersonal credibility (with their offspring). Parents must decide whether to focus on their teens' driving, drinking, diet, drugs, exercise, hygiene, studies, friends, sports, volunteering, moods, allergies, or physical safety, among other things. Within options potentially under their control, parents, too, must decide whether to invest in problem-focused interventions (e.g., grounding, curfews, driver education) or youth development ones (e.g., home schooling, family activities, religion).

Overview

The choices that policy makers and parents make or advocate reflect some amalgam of their values (about what matters) and beliefs (about what works). This paper casts these youth-specific choices in the general terms of priority-setting research and practice. One goal of these general approaches is increasing the expected value of invested resources. A second is clarifying the roles of social policy and social science in decision making, both for choices that have become norms and for new proposals. A third goal is revealing the value assumptions embedded in ostensibly objective analyses, clarifying the extent to which their conclusions are predetermined by their framing. For example, analyses focused on problematic end states (e.g., risk behaviors, adverse health outcomes) can divert attention from common sources, which contribute to multiple end states without being the primary determinant of any (e.g., low literacy, low birthweight). End-state analyses also divert attention from any value that programs have, independent of their effects on risk outcomes, such as making a social statement or contributing to those who implement them. Abstinence programs and Drug Abuse Resistance Education (D.A.R.E.), for example, might be rationally justified on those grounds, even if they had little direct effect on teens' sexuality or drug use. Whether they should be depends on what one values.

The next section, "Structuring Prioritization," introduces some general concepts and nomenclature. The following section, "Social Mechanisms for Priority Setting," contrasts two general approaches to determining priorities, differing in how explicitly they address value issues. The next section, "Deliberative Mechanisms for Priority Setting," considers ways to determine the relevant values, with particular reference to analogous processes developed for setting environment priorities, over the past generation. The "Conclusion" speculates on the circumstances under which deliberate prioritization might and should occur.

STRUCTURING PRIORITIZATION

Trying to Separate Facts and Values

Implicitly or explicitly, any policy regarding adolescent welfare embodies some notion of the overall burden that teens bear and its various expressions. These notions are reflected in the overall resources that teen issues receive and their allocation across problems. Pursued deliberately, the risk-assessment process has two stages: (1) characterizing the set of relevant adolescent vulnerabilities and (2) deciding what importance (or "weight") to assign to each threat (see Chapter 5 Annex). The first stage is largely a matter of scientific fact, the second largely a matter of values.

This fact/value distinction was central to the National Research Council's (1983) "red book," a founding document of risk assessment. Research and experience have shown life and analysis to be more complicated than this seemingly tidy separation suggests (e.g., Crouch and Wilson, 1981; Fischhoff et al., 1981; Institute of Medicine, 1998, 1999; National Research Council, 1996). Nonetheless, it is a point of departure for translating adolescent concerns into risk-based terms. These terms may have value in their own right, as a way of clarifying the structure of choices (complementing comprehensive analyses, such as Blum et al., this volume, and Burt et al., this volume). They may also help to make the case for youth when health and policy debates are cast in risk terms (as may happen increasingly).

In the first stage, conventional scientific procedures are used to estimate the impacts on teens associated with different conditions. The application (and review) of these procedures should follow accepted scientific practice. However, doing so inevitably requires making value-laden assumptions, when the terms of the research are specified and its results are interpreted. These assumptions need to be determined explicitly, lest the values be hidden under a guise of analytic objectivity, or buried even more deeply in priorities arising from unstructured group processes or individual ruminations. The formalisms of risk assessment are intended to accomplish this task by making all steps in the prioritization process explicit and subject to external review.

Nonetheless, any procedure, formal or otherwise, affords an advantage to those having greater fluency in its application. Indeed, much of the opposition to risk-based decision making in other areas reflects a fear that the promise of openness will not be realized. Rather, a new cadre of technical specialists will interject themselves in the process. Risk analyses can, in principle, consider a broad set of considerations without the sometimes-controversial monetization required by economic analyses (the primary current form of integrative approach). However, that promise will not be realized if the analyses are impenetrable to nonspecialists. One hope of this exposition is to clarify the assumptions made in prioritization, however it is accomplished.

What Might Matter?

The first of those assumptions is which things to consider. Box 5-1 shows three widely distributed sets of measures, translated from the originals so that all indicators are formulated negatively. The first list, from *Healthy People 2010*, has primarily health effects and (fairly proximal) predisposing conditions. The former are relatively uncontroversial, as outcomes that any society would want to avoid—even if there are disagreements about the completeness of the set and the weight to assign its members. The latter are more problematic. These conditions could be justified as indicators because they lead to adverse outcomes, a scientific claim. If those outcomes are also on the first list, then including the predisposing conditions would represent double counting. On the other hand, these conditions might efficiently represent a suite of concerns that are hard to assess directly (e.g., the variety of respiratory effects associated with airborne particulates). If so, then they might both avoid double counting and draw needed attention to problems with diffuse effects.

However, placing a predisposing condition on the list also may reflect a value judgment, in the sense of its being considered bad, regardless of any associated health effects. For example, "irresponsible" sexual behavior may be treated as offensive, even if it does not lead to sexually transmitted diseases or undesired pregnancies. Such values should be reflected in the weights assigned to the different measures. Continuing the example, irresponsible sex should receive extra weight from individuals who are offended by the act, as well as being worried about the health outcomes it can cause.[1]

Thus, even this simple list could reflect rather different rationales. The reference document (Department of Health and Human Services, 2000) describes the extensive consultation process that led to selecting these indicators (11,000 public comments are still available at http://*www.health.gov/healthypeople/*), as well as the comprehensiveness of its view (467 objectives, organized into 28 focus areas). This very sweep led to a search for leading indicators that would focus attention. That selection process was guided by the indicators' "ability to motivate action, the availability of data to mea-

[1]Depending on the intent of the list's compilers, everything but violence and injury could be considered a predisposing condition, in the sense of increasing the risk of some health problem. Indeed, even these two entries could serve that role, as when violent injuries (e.g., sexual assault) precipitate mental health problems.

sure their progress, and their relevance as broad public health issues" (p. 24). Thus, the task force considered both science (what will work) and values (what matters).

The report does not say how to resolve conflicts when initiatives directed at different problems compete for limited funds. Being on the list is, therefore, necessary, but not sufficient, for securing resources. The document assigns a "key role [to] community partnerships" for setting actual priorities (and implementing them) (DHHS, 2000, p. 4). However, limited guidance is provided for how such partnerships are to reach those priorities. As a result, prioritization is left to group (or political) processes: who gets to the table; who controls the agenda; who summarizes the proceedings. Stopping at this point may be entirely appropriate for these topics and the role of a federal agency. However, it leaves the process incomplete. Some of the approaches described here may be useful to those empowered to complete the work.

Deliberately Embedding Values in a Method

One place in which *Healthy People 2010* does attempt to direct the process is in measuring those outcomes that a prioritizing group decides to value. It makes "eliminate health disparities" one of its two overarching goals, on a par with "increase the quality and years of healthy life." It supports that focus by representing disparities in some of its measures (e.g., access to health care among different populations). Aggregate measures do not distinguish who suffers from a problem or benefits from a solution. Arguably, a life is a life and a cough is a cough, regardless of who suffers. However, ethical cases have been made for various forms of differential weighting. One common proposal assigns added weight to improvements benefiting individuals exposed to risks involuntarily (Lowrance, 1975; Starr, 1969). Those individuals might have been born with a problem or have had no political or economic influence over the conditions that created it. Involuntarily assumed risks also may have fewer compensating benefits (compared to risks that people chose to bring on themselves). Weighting involuntary risks more heavily provides a way to address such inequities.

It is also possible to value the people affected by risks differentially because of who they are, rather than what they have done—or have had done to them. Some such weighting inevitably is embedded in the procedures of any priority scheme. For example, mortality risk may be measured in terms of probability of death from each source being considered, or in

BOX 5-1
Alternative Indicators of Adolescent Vulnerability

Healthy People 2010: Leading Health Indicators (DHHS, 2000)

Outcomes
- Tobacco use
- Substance abuse
- Mental health problems
- Injury and violence

Predisposing Conditions
- Overweight and obesity
- Physical inactivity
- Irresponsible sexual behavior
- Environmental pollution
- Lack of immunization
- Limited access to health care

America's Children

Outcomes
- Poor health
- Chronic health conditions limiting activity
- Mortality
- Child bearing
- Cigarette smoking
- Alcohol use
- Substance abuse
- Victim of violent crime
- Abuse and neglect

Predisposing Conditions
- Poverty
- Food insecurity

terms of lost life expectancy arising from those deaths. Considering the number of years lost with each death puts a premium on deaths among young people. Using it focuses attention on threats that disproportionately affect them, such as accidents, relative to diseases of the aged, such as arte-

Housing problems
Parental employment insecurity
Lacking health insurance
Difficulty speaking English
Lacking math and reading proficiency
Neither working nor in school

UN Convention on the Rights of the Child

Outcomes
Nondiscrimination
Survival and development
Name and nationality
Preservation of identity
Contact with parents
Freedom of expression, thought, conscience, religion, and association
Privacy
Health
Standard of living adequate for physical, mental, spiritual, moral, and social development
Protection from drug abuse, sexual exploitation, abduction, torture, and armed conflicts
Leisure

Predisposing Conditions
Decisions made in the best interests of the child
Access to information
Special protection for refugees, disabled, adopted, without families, and minorities
Health and social services
Education developing personality, talents, and mental and physical abilities
Age-appropriate justice, promoting sense of dignity and worth

riosclerosis. Of course, focusing on deaths raises the profile of risks such as auto accidents relative to ones that cause mostly morbidity and misery (such as drugs). Whatever unit is used, it represents a value (even if that choice is made unwittingly).

The second list, created by the Federal Interagency Forum on Child and Family Statistics (1997), also includes both outcomes and predisposing conditions. Compared with *Healthy People 2010,* it has a larger set of health outcomes, while still not subsuming the previous list (e.g., mental health problems, unintentional injury). One could ask whether the compilers of the first list were not interested in activities limited by chronic health conditions (a value question) or believed that these outcomes were predicted from others in their list (a scientific question). As with the first list, the Predisposing Conditions also could be viewed as negative ends in their own right. Were that the case, then the second list would represent a broader definition of the conditions that our society owes its citizens. If not, then including these additional conditions reflects an alternative view of the facts regarding predisposing causes, with a larger role assigned to social and economic factors, such an employment and housing status.[2]

Evidence-Driven Criteria

The third set of criteria is taken from an international document, the United Nations (UN) Convention on the Rights of the Child (signed by all member countries except Somalia, which lacks a central government, and the United States). One obligation of signing countries is to compile statistics reporting on the state of their children, reflecting these concerns. Perhaps the most striking difference between this list and its predecessors is the emphasis on political rights. In Box 5-1, some of these are cast as outcomes, others as predisposing conditions (a distinction that we imposed on the Convention's list). In the former role, these criteria are ends in themselves; in the latter, they are means to other ends. Reasonable individuals could disagree about these roles, and about the kinds of evidence needed to evaluate the importance of each. For example, one might consider any discrimination to be wrong or only discrimination that could be linked to end states, such as survival and development. In the latter case, the weight assigned to discrimination would depend on the strength of the demonstrated connection (as determined, perhaps, by the sort of root-cause analyses demonstrated by Blum et al., this volume, and Burt et al., this volume).

[2]Their omission from the first list could reflect a value judgment, to the effect that these conditions are predictors of the health outcomes, but not ones that should concern anyone other than the individuals involved.

Neglecting discrimination, in the absence of such evidence, need not reflect indifference to this aspect of young people's fate. Rather, the ties with direct effects may seem sufficiently strong that it is better to measure them than discrimination. Doing so avoids double counting (both causes and effects). Effects may be more observable and less controversial. One also may feel that discrimination is a separate effect, but belongs to some other jurisdiction, and hence is not an aspect of adolescent health and safety. The impact of that claim depends on whether the other jurisdiction actually assumes responsibility for assessing, and addressing, discrimination—and on whether it is, in fact, a problem. The UN Convention criteria are meant to serve the interests of young people in widely varying circumstances around the world. Problems that are egregious in some countries may be minor in other, more fortunate ones (e.g., in which few children are denied names or nationalities).

At least two of the UN criteria should discourage the adoption of measures that obscure disparities when looking at overall performance. One is discrimination, which might predict such disparities. The second is special protection for several inherently vulnerable populations. Without those protections, one might presume variation in the achievement of other criteria, even without assessing it.

Another apparent difference in the UN Convention criteria is the inclusion of such "positive" criteria such as education developing personality, talents, and mental and physical abilities. Like nondiscrimination, these criteria might be treated as ends or means. A society may be held to fail its children, if they fail to achieve their full potential. Or, the lack of effective investment in development may provide a predictor of other valued criteria. Like nondiscrimination, such education may be ignored because it belongs to another jurisdiction or because it is too hard to measure. Doing so requires an explicit theory for how various kinds and quantities of education achieve desired results. Where such measures of positive contribution are lacking, one might have to revert to the deficit model underlying most criteria.

Criteria for Criteria

The empirical constraints on measurement feature centrally in the selection rules described as guiding the choice of measures in *America's Children*:

- *Easy to understand* by broad audiences.
- *Objectively* based on substantial research connecting them to child well-being and based on *reliable* data.
- *Balanced* so that no single area of children's lives dominates the report.
- *Measured regularly* so that they can be updated and show trends over time.
- *Representative* of large segments of the population, rather than one particular group.

Such practically oriented rules have significant, perhaps obvious, strengths and weaknesses. Easily understood measures can capture the popular imagination, mobilizing appropriate concern for young people. However, they can crowd out more subtle measures and may be "understood" in ways different from the applicable science. For example, the emerging interest in resilience (Masten, 2001) reflects a perception that apparently transparent deficit measures (showing how teens were damaged or what they could not do and did wrong) created an incomplete, misleading picture of development.

It is hard to argue with objective measurement, nor with having a strong research basis. However, standards of "objectivity" vary across disciplines, running the risk of capture by a particular perspective. In the present context, there might be a preference for standardized measures, suited to survey administration or data mining from public health records. That would come at the expense of more intense observation of individual young people (Kubey et al., 1996). The yield from such measures could, in principle, compensate for the lower reliability and smaller samples (due to more expensive measurement). However, that is not a simple argument, especially when it needs to be sufficiently persuasive to overcome accepted practices—and when change would disrupt the continuity of an established data set (however imperfect it might be).

There is a natural appeal to seeking a balance, across the areas of children's lives, and representativeness, across the children being studied. These default assumptions render no child and no problem more important than any other. However, as mentioned, one of the earliest lessons in the development of risk assessment was that "a death is a death" is not an ethically neutral position. In the context of adolescent welfare and vulnerability, equal representation means, for example, assigning no special weight to the fate of teens from particularly challenged backgrounds (such as those cited for special protection in the UN Convention). Even if differential weighting is inappropriate, a case still might be made for differential sampling, so as to increase the statistical power of attempts to understand the status of focal populations. For example, the 1997 National Longitudinal Study of Youth (Bureau of Labor Statistics, 1998) oversamples African American and Hispanic teens in order to understand better their status and its determinants. That strategy increases the chances of discovering risk factors and documenting them with the precision needed to drive social policy.

The appropriateness of having a balanced set of criteria depends on which areas are included and how they are categorized. Balance might be a charade if one believed that important domains have been ignored (e.g., predisposing causes, psychological impacts, political rights). Balanced attention to measures would not mean equal attention to problems if some areas were treated in much greater detail that others. That might happen for justifiable reasons (e.g., there are many different problems, with relatively distinct etiology, under "infectious diseases") or more questionable ones (e.g., there are many more scientists working in one area who have had time to develop a larger suite of measures). Whether it leads to appropriate attention is partly a matter of values (does this form of balance reflect the weight that the problems deserve?) and partly a matter of science (do the selected measures capture their respective domains equally well?).

SOCIAL MECHANISMS FOR PRIORITY SETTING

Thus, these ambitious efforts to characterize threats to young people (and signs of well-being) are necessary, but not sufficient for setting priorities. Without measures, and the analysis that went into their creation and collection, there would be little systematic evidence to justify or allay concerns. However, both the selection and formulation of measures are value laden, in the sense of highlighting particular problems and specific formulations of them. Without an orderly process of selecting and applying values, one cannot know whether society is acting appropriately in its relative response to particular problems or its overall response to the burden on youth (as determined by aggregating across individual problems).

In principle, there are two ways of determining values. They are the methods of *revealed preferences,* looking at past behaviors, and *expressed preferences,* looking at current attitudes (Bentkover et al., 1985). Their respective strengths and weaknesses, in general, are well known (and might seem obvious, were it not the case that each family of methods had such strong adherents and detractors).

Revealed Preferences

When people take action (including deliberate inaction), their behaviors reflect a willingness to accept the associated consequences (e.g., economic, social, psychological). That prospect should increase their investment in the decision-making process: how hard they think, how vigorously they collect data, how conscientiously they monitor subsequent developments. Unfortunately, without some independent assessment, action alone does not guarantee that people have understood the facts of a situation nor the implications of their own values for it. Substantial literatures document the potential fallibility of people's judgments of facts and the malleability of their values (when people must articulate the implications of their basic values in novel situations) (e.g., Dawes and Hastie, 2001; Kahneman et al., 1982; McFadden, 1999). Thus, people's choices may not reflect their preferences.

Even when choices are made under favored circumstances (with clear, informed thought), it can be difficult to discern the values they express. Economists, in particular, have developed sophisticated procedures for answering the question "why did they do that?", suited to situations involving multiple decisions of a single type (each characterized by the same set of features). Nonetheless, even when they have been applied rigorously and have demonstrated their predictive ability in new situations, these equations have some inherent limits (Dawes, 1979). These include partitioning the importance attributed to related factors (multicollinearity) and determining whether predictors are the true drivers of behavior, or merely surrogates (when the two factors might denote rather different values).

Such analytical procedures are most comfortably applied to discerning the preferences revealed in choices among goods traded in properly functioning markets. Such markets have well-informed consumers, making free choices among options that offer the range of tradeoffs possible with existing technology (broadly defined to include both social and engineering knowledge). For example, some people buy presweetened cereals made from heavily refined grains, despite having whole-grain alternatives in close proximity and sugar packages on an aisle that they pass anyway. If the conventional assumptions hold, one might conclude that they prefer the taste and texture of refined grains, and prefer to pay the premium for presweetening (compared to adding the same amount of sugar at the table).

Potential Failures of Revelation

Those conclusions are threatened when competitive market assumptions are violated. Imperfect markets can result from informational failures (when the parties to a transaction have inaccurate or unequal knowledge) and institutional ones (e.g., externalities, restraints on trade). In the example given, informational failures can arise when consumers do not know the nutritional advantages of whole grain and cannot infer them from the aggregate information on the standard label (which reflects all ingredients). The weight of the sugar is listed explicitly; however, many consumers would be hardpressed to set up and execute the calculations needed to estimate the cost premium for presweetening. Even if they could determine the implications of their choices, many consumers might not think it was worth the effort. That might reflect an accurate assessment of the *transaction costs* of running the numbers, compared to the expected return on that effort (including how accurately it will be done and how big a signal it will reveal). Or, it might reflect misinformation (perhaps abetted by advertising and packaging) or failure to think at all. Or, it might reflect a preference for making the children happy (or quiet), in which case nutrition plays little role in the buyer's choice. In another context, debate rages over whether labeling foods containing genetically modified grains would provide consumers with vital information or misinform them by suggesting a nonexistent risk.

Inferring preferences from choices is also compromised by imperfections in the options available. For example, convenience stores sell only the most popular brands, limiting immediate choices and strengthening the market position of those brands (by increasing their economies of scale and providing the advertising of product placement). Even large stores vary widely in whether they provide more nutritious (or organic) foods, perhaps reflecting consumer preferences, perhaps suppressing them. Anything that reduces the availability of an option increases its cost and price, thereby raising the strength of preference needed to make the choice. Any market responds more to those with more money to spend, increasing the chances that they will find the desired options, with adequate accompanying information. Deliberate restraint of trade can further reduce options, as can imperfect research, development, and marketing processes—revealed when a seemingly obvious product reaches the market, long after it was technologically feasible.

Social Revelation

Similar, and additional, complications arise when preferences are sought in collective actions. Thus, for example, in an ideal political system, government spending would reflect the preferences of a well-informed electorate, with each citizen receiving equal weight. The multiple failures in these processes are well known among those interested in such things (even if they disagree about sources and solutions). One possible reflection of the efficacy of political processes is seen in analyses of the amounts of money spent per life saved in different domains. Other things being equal, these amounts should be the same. If one program can save twice as many lives as another, for the same investment, then the money should be transferred there (as a "better buy" in life saving). However, analyses have shown wide disparities in the efficacy of programs (e.g., Tengs et al., 1995).

If one accepts these estimates of dollars spent and lives saved, then these programs do not reveal a consistent societal preference of willingness to pay for life saving. It is difficult to say, then, what they do reveal. One claim is that they reflect stable public values applied consistently to risk perceptions that vary widely in their accuracy (e.g., Breyer, 1993; Cohen and Lee, 1979). According to such claims, the public is disproportionately alarmed about some risks, forcing government and industry to pay disproportionate amounts for their control—consuming resources that would be better spent on controlling other risks (or on other social purposes). Unfortunately, there is rarely the evidence needed to evaluate rigorously the accuracy of these claims and the associated public perceptions (Fischhoff, 1999, 2000; Fischhoff et al., 1997; Lichtenstein et al., 1978; Millstein and Halpern-Felsher, this volume). Nor are there concrete plans for ensuring the transfer of funds to more efficient methods of risk reduction.

As a result, many other interpretations are possible. One is that the political system reveals consistent, informed beliefs that define the benefits of programs more broadly than "expected lives saved." Citizens might, legitimately, care about reduced morbidity, enhanced resilience, and better education, not to mention the impacts of programs on citizen participation, economic development, and public morality (however defined), among other possible concerns. Unless they are guaranteed the fungibility of funds, from less efficient to more efficient ways of serving public needs, citizens might refuse to cede any protections. However, these programs could just as well reflect the net impact of political processes having little to do with citizen concerns (e.g., lobbying, concessions made in trade negotiations, payoffs among legislative committee chairs, litigation).

Even within the domain of professionally managed, health-focused actions, the preferences revealed in actions can be obscure. For example, in 1998, Congress made the reauthorization of the National Institutes of Health (NIH) contingent on its adoption of an explicit procedure for prioritizing its expenditures. In the associated political debate, one form of evidence used to substantiate claims of incoherent expenditures was the ratio of dollars spent to deaths for various health problems. In this light, it was argued that HIV/AIDS received disproportionate resources. NIH's (1998) response was that it followed a multiattribute approach to prioritization, considering factors such as consequences other than mortality, the losses associated with each death (as a quality adjusted life years [QALY] or disability adjusted life years [DALY] evaluations might try to capture), the opportunities for scientific progress, and the importance of research results for other problems. As a step toward applying these criteria more explicitly, NIH adopted one recommendation of an Institute of Medicine (1998) panel—creating a Council of Public Representatives to understand public preferences more directly.

Social Obstacles to Preference Revelation

As in markets for public goods, a natural advantage often accrues to those "good causes" that already have market share. They develop a cadre of supporters and dependents who will work to support existing programs—sometimes even if they have no demonstrated efficacy or inefficacy. The scientists working on these programs are more likely to have their own dedicated study sections (for evaluating proposals), training grants, fundamentally sympathetic journals, and opportunities to observe fortuitous interesting results. Studied problems are also more likely to have the large data sets that facilitate demonstrating their magnitude and progress. Thus, past preferences shape future preferences by keeping attention on traditional problems.

These challenges to inferring preferences from actions arise (in one form or another) whether the currency is program expenditures, philanthropic contributions, or volunteering time. The limits to relying on revealed preferences can be seen in the periodic realization that an issue has been badly neglected, relative to investments in related issues. Women's health, child abuse and neglect, and positive youth development are among the latent issues that have emerged over the past two decades, the importance of which was not revealed in existing funding priorities (Lerner, in press). It would not be hard to propose potential biases in these processes, which might be used to correct observed preferences. For example, Burt et al. (this volume) argue that "tangible" immediate effects of adolescents' problems (e.g., juvenile justice, remedial education, chronic health, social assistance) are overemphasized, relative to "intangible" later costs (e.g., lost human potential). Doing so would mean moving away from being guided by revealed preferences to using them as an anchor upon which to base expressed preferences. It would mean concluding that we are not getting it right and need some direct intervention to set our priorities straight.

DELIBERATIVE MECHANISMS FOR PRIORITY SETTING

Expressed Preferences

Studies asking people for their values can, in principle, overcome some of these difficulties. Properly designed studies can explain the issues in ways that improve participants' understanding. They can present alternative perspectives and help people to triangulate among them so that they can articulate the implications of their basic values for particular situations. Such studies can specify the exact issues that concern policy makers, as well as pose alternative ones. For that to happen, the studies need to attend to each stage of the design process: (1) characterizing the risks in common terms; (2) communicating those risks to the individuals doing the evaluation; and (3) allowing the evaluators to articulate and express their preferences.

This section considers the challenges facing the execution of each stage, illustrated by an approach developed in the Department of Engineering and Public Policy at Carnegie Mellon University (Fischhoff, 1995; Morgan et al., 1996). It was developed in response to a request from the Office of Science and Technology Policy for a way to set risk priorities that would meet the following criteria: (1) reflect the multiattribute character of risk; (2) ensure that participants understood the facts of their tasks; (3) reveal the logic of the expressed preferences; and (4) allow comparisons (and the search for consistency) across programs and agencies (Davies, 1996). We have considerable experience with this approach, as well as studies evaluating its reliability and validity (Florig et al., in press; Morgan et al., in press).

However, it is used here not to advocate its adoption, but to demonstrate the functions that any comprehensive approach to prioritization will have to fulfill, one way or another. Fortuitously for the present context, although originally concerned with environmental risks, we developed and tested the method with an experimental test bed dedicated to risks to children in schools. It was intended to provide study participants with a familiar setting and take advantage of statistics compiled in one of the last reports from the Office of Technology Assessment (1995). Sadly, schools provide a sufficiently diverse set of risks to test the generality of any method. Stimulus material characterizing risks at the hypothetical Centerville Middle School can be found at http://www.epp.cmu.edu/research/EPP_risk.html.[3]

Characterizing Risks

Priorities should be based on the best available technical information, but without having the data analyses prejudge value issues (in any of the ways discussed earlier). Leaving all the analytical options open can, however, result in an incomprehensible deluge of statistics showing every conceivable way of looking at the problem. One procedure for reducing the set of possibilities is identifying features that vary so little across the risks that they could not affect priorities. For example, threatening national security is an important feature, in the abstract, but not an issue for middle schools (unless, perhaps, they have an extraordinary cadre of hackers).[4]

Another approach is to take advantage of the empirical correlations among those features that do vary across the risks. Many studies (reviewed most recently by Jenni, 1997) have asked people to rate multiple hazards on various features, typically finding that two or three factors suffice to explain most of the variance in the ratings. Slovic (1987) calls these factors *knowledge, dread,* and *number.* Knowledge includes whether the risk is old,

[3]It includes blueprints of each floor, a perspective drawing of school grounds, and a map of the town showing the location of CMS and risk-relevant features (e.g., fire department, highway, railroad tracks).

[4]Graduate apartments are a popular topic for stimuli in choice experiments conducted by graduate students. Those students have considerable expertise in the topic and can get their friends to serve as expert subjects. At times, these studies find that cost is unimportant to grad students—because the options have been restricted to the narrow price range that is feasible with grad stipends. Under that constraint, other factors (e.g., location, noise level) predominate.

familiar, and understood by science, as well as whether it produces effects that are immediate, observable, and known to those exposed. Dread includes whether risks are uncontrollable, catastrophic, global, fatal, inequitably distributed, not easily reduced, increasing over time, involuntary, personal or affect future generations,. Number includes the extent of individual and population risks of death and injury. It is not hard to see how risks high on many of these properties also might be high on others in the same factors.

Where these correlations hold, a factor could, in effect, be represented by any feature that loads heavily on it. We chose two features for each factor, both to give a richer feeling for its domain and to allow evaluators to choose the feature they found most meaningful. For example, old technologies tend to be understood better by science. However, somewhat different values are invoked by judging a risk more harshly because it is new and because it is understood poorly. For each factor, we chose features according to their comprehensibility, normative status, and supporting data. Knowledge was represented by "quality of scientific understanding" and "time between exposure and health effects"; dread by "greatest number of deaths in a single episode" and "ability of student/parent to control exposure"; and number by mortality and morbidity. To reduce framing effects (Kahneman and Tversky, 1979; Schwarz, 1999), we represented mortality risk in two formally equivalent measures: "number of deaths per year" and the "chance in a million of death per year for the average student." To capture potential disparities in exposure, we included the "chance in a million of death per year for the student at highest risk." We broke morbidity into four components, reflecting severity and duration. We represented the substantial uncertainties in the quantitative attributes with low, high, and best estimates. Finally, we created a composite attribute of "combined uncertainty in death, illness, and injury" by taking the mean of the geometric standard deviations of the mortality and morbidity attributes. Overall, this meant 11 independent attributes, not counting the 2 formats for mortality. An example appears in Box 5-2 (which is explained below).

Characterizing risks in terms of a common set of features creates a level playing field among them, in a way that is subject to public review. However, as discussed, doing so is only one element of task specification that can affect the resulting priorities (and actions following from them). Florig et al. (in press) discuss other design choices in creating our experimental test bed, as well as how they may have affected priorities. Our choices include:

BOX 5-2
Example of a Risk-Summary Brochure Displaying the Risk Attributes

School Bus Accidents

Summary:
Most school bus-related deaths occur among students who are outside the bus either getting on or getting off. Half of school bus injuries occur among students on the bus. At Centerville Middle School half of the 430 students ride the school bus, almost identical to the national average. Accidents involving more than one death are very rare. Because CMS buses use the Alvarez Expressway and cross the C&LL rail line, the risk of a catastrophic bus accident in Centerville is estimated to be between four and six times higher than the national average.

School bus accident risk for Centerville Middle School*

Student deaths	*Low estim.*	***Best estimate***	*High estim.*
Number of deaths per year	.0001	**.0002**	.0004
Chance in a million of death per year for the average student	.25	**0.5**	1
Chance in a million of death per year for the student at highest risk	0.5	**1**	2
Greatest number of deaths in a single episode		**20 - 50**	
Student illness or injury			
More serious long-term cases per year	.0002	**.0006**	.002
Less serious long-term cases per year	.0004	**.0015**	.004
More serious short-term cases per year	.001	**.002**	.006
Less serious short-term cases per year	.002	**.005**	.015
Other Factors			
Time between exposure and health effects		**immediate**	
Quality of scientific understanding		**high**	
Combined uncertainty in death, illness, injury		**0.5 (low)**	
Ability of student/parent to control exposure		**moderate**	

*See "Notes on the Numbers" for definitions and explanations of assumptions.

SOURCE: Carnegie Mellon University (2001).

BOX 5-3
Risks Evaluated in Centerville Middle School: Risk-Ranking Tested

Accidental injuries (excluding sports)
Airplane crashes
Allergens in indoor air
Asbestos

Bites and stings
Building collapse

Common infectious diseases
Commuting to school on foot, by bike, or by car

Drowning

Electric and magnetic fields from electric power
Electric shock

Fire and explosion
Food poisoning

Hazardous materials transport

Intentional injury
Injury or harm; self-inflicted

Lead poisoning
Less common infectious diseases
Lightning

Radon gas

School bus accidents

Team sports

• We sought a broad set of risks (see Box 5-3), each having morbidity or mortality potential, resulting in a range of outcomes that is narrower, but easier to characterize than those proposed by Burt et al. (this volume).

• We grouped risks according to potential interventions (e.g., separating accidents into falls, sports, school buses, and commuting in private vehicles because interventions for each category lie in different jurisdictions).

• When a risk (e.g., driving) had both proximal sources (e.g., drinking and driving) and predisposing ones (e.g., alcoholism), we focused on the former, given the stronger evidence for the linkage and lines of responsibility for action.

• We omitted risks of inaction (e.g., not having effective programs to keep kids in school or to discourage risk behaviors, such as smoking and physical inactivity) because of their diffuse effects and sources.

• We made no distinctions among students beyond their risk levels (partially captured by the contrast between risk to the average and the most exposed student).

- We restricted risk estimates to direct effects on students in the school, even when indirect effects are likely (e.g., transmission of infectious disease to siblings, emotional suffering among parents of injured students, worrying by parents when children are exposed to risks). The analyses by Blum et al. (this volume) and Burt et al. (this volume) suggest alternative conceptualizations.

Risk Communication

The suite of data needed to do these issues justice creates a significant cognitive challenge for the evaluators, who must both take it all in and overcome potential pitfalls in their own judgmental processes. Our approach addresses these issues in both how information is communicated and how individuals are led through it. This section discusses our communication strategies.

At the most prosaic level, we took advantage of research in document design (e.g., Schriver, 1989) to create an accessible layout, the first page of which appears in Box 5-2. Within it, information is organized in brief, conceptually distinct units intended to allow approaching information for different purposes. The top of the first page identifies the risk category (e.g., school bus accidents), followed by a one-paragraph description further defining it and roughly indicating its magnitude for several risk attributes. The remainder of the page presents the summary table. The second page provides a general discussion, including what is known and uncertain regarding each attribute. The third page begins with qualitative and quantitative discussions of the risk at the school. It includes comparisons with typical schools and homes, as well as government standards (e.g., the Environmental Protection Agency's 4-picoCurie-per-liter-action-limit)—taking care not to give these comparisons any rhetorical force (so that participants feel free to apply their own standards). The brochure concludes with the actions that the school has taken regarding the risk, in order to (1) provide a realistic context; (2) focus on residual risks; and (3) distinguish risks from the feasibility or cost of risk management. Supplementary documents were available on site, elaborating on the information in the summary sheets and documenting their sources.

The wording of the brochures used simple, nontechnical language. Where possible, it took advantage of existing research on risk communication to improve comprehension (e.g., Fischhoff, 1999; Millstein and Halpern-Felsher, this volume; Morgan et al., 2001). The explanations of the phenomena were intended to provide participants with an intuitive, qualitative feel for the processes determining the quantitative levels of risk being described—as well as a feeling of empowerment for making these choices. Risks were expressed numerically to avoid the ambiguity of verbal quantifiers (e.g., Budescu and Wallsten, 1995). Terms known to lack clear, consensual definitions were avoided or defined (e.g., McIntyre and West, 1993). Successive drafts were evaluated with think-aloud protocols. Different individuals had ultimate editorial authority for the accuracy of the science and the appropriateness of the language. This division of labor was intended to avoid the stylistic incoherence and endless editing possible when anyone in the process feels entitled to tinker with the text.

Once risk estimates are individually comprehensible, participants must compare them. The brochure's design was intended to facilitate sorting, shuffling, and categorizing. We also provided a large (28 cm × 43 cm) chart ranking the 22 risks according to each attribute. It allowed easy determination of relative rankings on any attribute, and showed how risks high on one attribute might be low on another.

Our goal was to ensure that risk rankers have an accurate, consensual understanding of the issues facing them, even if they choose to disagree about their resolution. Procedures exist for measuring the accuracy of the resultant understanding (Fischhoff et al., 1997). The adequacy of that understanding depends on the sensitivity of the task at hand. Sometimes, even a rough understanding of risks will allow distinguishing among them. Sometimes, greater precision is required.

Articulating Values

Once risks have been understood, setting priorities among them faces several challenges. One is the continuing cognitive load of keeping them in mind, even with aids like the brochures and summary sheets. The second is individuals' need to articulate values for these specific questions, consistent with their basic values on the general issues. The third challenge is that when people lack prepared answers to a question, they can be subject to *framing effects,* such that ostensibly equivalent ways of posing questions can lead to different answers. Alternative frames may prime different values or suggest different investigator expectations. The fourth challenge is that individual values are often socially determined, in the sense that people want to know what others think, reflecting their personal values and life experiences. The fifth is that any attempt to derive group values runs the risk of poorly mediated group processes suppressing some views and giving undue weight to others.

We designed the following process as a way to address these concerns: Individuals receive the risk summary information before their initial group meeting, with instructions to study it and reach tentative opinions. After that study, but before any group discussion, each participant evaluates the risks. Doing so is intended to help them to articulate their own values—and emphasize their legitimacy, independent of what is expressed in group discussions. These evaluations are done in two ways, intended to provide alternative perspectives on the issues and reduce the effects of any initial frame. One is *holistic,* the other *analytic.* The former has them rank the risks directly. The latter uses a simplified multiattribute procedure: participants rate the risk attributes in terms of relative importance, which the moderators convert into implied risk rankings. When the holistic and analytic rankings diverge, participants are encouraged to reflect on the reasons and seek reconciliation.

The ensuing group discussions are moderated to facilitate sharing perspectives and helping participants to articulate their opinions. Group size is set large enough to reduce any individual's influence, but small enough to facilitate group discussion. The length of the discussion depends on the complexity of the issues and its fruitfulness.[5] Consensus is sought as a way to focus the deliberations, but not forced, explicitly recognizing that there may be differences of opinion that a successful process will bring into focus. Toward the end, the holistic and analytic individual evaluations are repeated, both to create a record of those beliefs and to recognize further their legitimacy (e.g., for individuals who are reluctant to express their views publicly).

These discussions about the importance of risks often evoke concerns about the feasibility and cost of strategies for managing them (as might individual deliberations). Both the initial instructions and subsequent re-

[5]One device that we have used is to have the group sort the complete set of risk summary sheets into three piles representing high, medium, and low concern. Each pile is then ranked internally, after which the boundary members are compared (e.g., the lowest risks in the high pile and the highest ones in the medium pile). This procedure could be used, of course, to manage the cognitive load for individual rankers as well.

minders distinguish these issues, asking participants to focus on importance. These instructions acknowledge that large risks may be neglected if nothing can be done about them. However, recognizing that fact is important, especially if it reveals too little investment in developing solutions. Conversely, small risks may be addressed if there are efficient solutions. However, that might mean they have received disproportionate attention in the past. When participants raise issues related to solutions, those are duly noted, both to acknowledge their eventual importance and to help participants make the conceptual distinction.

Thus, the procedure allows participants to triangulate group and individual perspectives, as well as holistic and analytic ones. It also allows policy makers to use results in different ways. They can take initial values or concluding ones, group values or individual ones (collected in private). Policy makers can consider the change between initial and final values, individuals' agreement with other group members, the degree of consensus on particular risks (in absolute terms or relative to the general level of consensus), and the coherence between holistic and analytic values. That interpretation should depend on the circumstances. For example, a group's consensus may mean little unless its membership has some policy significance (e.g., an identifiable interest group, accustomed to resolving such issues together). Otherwise, it was just a vehicle for exposing individuals to diverse views. In conclusion, participants evaluate the process, including how well they communicated their views, as measures of its success (and legitimacy).

The summary sheet ranks the risks by individual attributes. Although presented as effort saving, these rankings also show simple policies that participants could choose to adopt. One also could present rankings that reflect other, more complex principles, saving the more complex mental arithmetic that each requires. Those principles might be derived from the professional literature, ethical analyses, citizen interviews, or government regulations. For example, they might present the estimated (public or private) economic burden of each risk (to the extent that it can be calculated). Presenting them reduces the risk of participants missing perspectives that they would value or executing them poorly. It increases the risk of biasing expressed preferences, if the offerings are unbalanced.

CONCLUSION

Although this chapter makes the case for setting priorities systematically, it also shows the challenges that such exercises face. Recognizing these challenges and possible ways to address them should improve the process. However, one still should ask whether the best possible *systematic* prioritization is advisable. It could fail a cost-effectiveness test, in the sense of being a poorer investment of management energy than the best possible *systemic* prioritization (focusing intently on whatever risks happen to draw one's attention). It could fail a cost-benefit test, in the sense of leaving one worse off than without any systematic analysis.

Many factors affect the relative efficacy of spreading a given amount of decision-making resources over the broad set of risks (ensuring that each gains some attention) or focusing it on the few risks that seize public (or agency) attention:

- How well is the overall world of risks understood? If relatively few risks have drawn any concerted attention, then it is more likely that resources have been misallocated, and a systematic review will be informative.
- How much can be learned from a relatively quick look at individual risks? If a serious examination is required to learn very much, then it is harder to justify a broad review.
- How likely is it that some risks have been systematically over- or underestimated (e.g., due to flawed reporting or analytical methods that emphasize particular concerns, perhaps ones that are quantified most easily)? Such suspicions increase the expected value of looking hard at those specific risks, rather than assuming that things are generally in order.
- How much precision is needed to move from risk ranking to option ranking? If regulatory constraints or political inertia require strong evidence, then focusing on specific risks becomes essential—even if a broader look might show that they are not the most important targets for that focus.
- How are risks prioritized—by a best guess or by a worst case estimate of their magnitude? A broad look might do more to shift the tails than the central tendencies of probability distributions over possible risk levels.

Bendor (1995) and Long and Fischhoff (2000) offer formal models for characterizing particular situations and simulating the expected yield of different strategies for prioritizing their risks. These models reflect concerns about the limits to analysis identified by Lindblom (1959), Simon (1957), and others. Even without running simulations, thinking about the formal properties of these situations should clarify what one wants, and can hope to get, from them. That assessment can be performed for the yield from both conventional procedures and more innovative ones. For example, our risk-ranking procedure is intended to increase the feasibility of systematic evaluation by using the time and energy of risk rankers more efficiently. Whether used on many risks or a few, such a procedure should increase the accountability of rankers by showing what evidence and factors have been considered (even if the integrative decision rule is embedded in their holistic judgments).

If prioritization means anything, it should be capable of changing resource allocations. Individuals concerned with teens' overall welfare should welcome an improvement in their ability to track the problems faced by teens (as a whole and by target subgroups). Such data should help to mobilize and allocate program resources. On the other hand, however valid the procedures, prioritization will tend to be opposed by individuals whose programs and concerns are relatively well supported—and to be endorsed by those who feel neglected. Analysis also can be used to frustrate and misdirect actions. "Further study" can be a ruse for protecting the status quo. Showing "better buys" in risk reduction is meaningless, or even disingenuous, unless there is a real opportunity to move funds from worse causes to better ones. When funds are not fungible, such comparisons can lead to canceling worthwhile programs without increasing support for better ones.[6]

Finally, some supporters and detractors of prioritization may be less concerned with adolescents than with how the choice of policy-making procedure affects civic governance. Policy-making procedures can range from direct democracy to having specialists act in the public's name without any consultation—arguing that they not only have a better command of the facts, but also a better understanding of what the public really wants. Toward the latter extreme, one finds metrics like QALYs (quality-adjusted life years) (Tengs and Wallace, 2000), which represent citizens' values by the views expressed by a one-time sample. Our own procedure lies further toward the former extreme, insofar as it allows the continuing involvement

[6]Kelman (cited in Kolata, 2001) recalls a meeting with EPA and NIH officials regarding the regulation of lead levels. "From my standpoint as a scientist, I realized that well nourished kids absorb less lead. So, being pretty naive, I said, 'Why not take the money that the EPA is talking about for lowering lead levels in drinking water and putting it into nourishing inner city kids?'" The EPA said it didn't feed children; the NIH said it didn't have the money. "It was a classic federal impasse . . . At which point I figured I'd better sit down and shut up."

of actual citizens, and not just summaries of their views. Thus, values shape both the priorities that we set on teens' welfare and the procedures that we use to reach those priorities—just as they, in turn, shape our future society.

ANNEX
SETTING PRIORITIES BY WEIGHTING ATTRIBUTES

The essence of priority setting is to identify the issues that matter, decide how important each is in the focal context, and then evaluate each option, considering how it stacks up on each issue, weighted by the relative importance of those issues. Multiattribute utility theory formalizes this logic (Fischhoff et al., 1984; Keeney and Raiffa, 1976; vonWinterfeldt and Edwards, 1986). In it, the issues are called *attributes* and relative importance is represented by *weights*. Although many sophisticated applications are possible, a weighted sum is adequate for characterizing options in many situations (Dawes, 1979).

In the case of adolescent well-being, the multiattribute degree of *concern* evoked by a source of vulnerability might be expressed as:

$$Concern_j = \sum_{i=1}^{n} w_i \times u_i(x_{ij})$$

where j is the source of vulnerability, i is an attribute, n is the number of attributes, w_i is the weight for attribute i, x_{ij} represents how source j performs in terms of attribute i, and u_i is the utility attached to that degree of attribute i.

This appendix illustrates how this approach might be applied to setting priorities. The rows of Table 5-1 list 12 attributes that might be considered when evaluating threats to the health and safety of students in a school. They include aspects of both mortality (number of deaths per year, average chance of death, highest chance of death for any student, and greatest number of deaths in a single episode) and morbidity (number of more and less serious cases of long- and short-term injuries and illnesses per year). The attributes also include features that often have been found to affect risk perceptions (e.g., Fischhoff et al., 1978; Morgan et al., in press; Slovic, 1987). These are the time between exposure and health effects, the quality of scientific understanding, the uncertainty regarding the outcomes, and the ability of students or parents to control exposure.

The columns of Table 5-1 show four weighting schemes that might be applied to these attributes. Set A reflects a person concerned only with the

TABLE 5-1 Four Possible Sets of Weights for 12 Attributes of Adolescent Vulnerability

	Importance Weighting Scheme			
Attribute	A	B	C	D
Number of deaths per year	0.050	0.050	0.050	0.150
Chance in a million of death per year for the average student	0.600	0.250	0.100	0.100
Chance in a million of death per year for the student at highest risk	0.300	0.250	0.100	0.100
Greatest number of deaths in a single episode	0.050	0.050	0.050	0.150
More serious long-term injuries or illnesses (cases per year)	0	0.200	0.150	0.025
Less serious long-term injuries or illnesses (cases per year)	0	0	0.200	0.025
More serious short-term injuries or illnesses (cases per year)	0	0.200	0.150	0.025
Less serious short-term injuries or illnesses (cases per year)	0	0	0.200	0.025
Time between exposure and health effects	0	0	0	0.100
Quality of scientific understanding	0	0	0	0.100
Uncertainty regarding death, illness, and injury	0	0	0	0.100
Ability of student/parent to control exposure	0	0	0	0.100
Sum of weights	1.000	1.000	1.000	1.000

probability of death. Set B corresponds to an individual concerned with serious illness and injury, as well as death. Set C weights also consider less serious illness and injury.[7] Finally, set D also pays attention to the "qualitative" aspects of the risk in the final four rows. Each set of weights has been normalized to total 1.0; they correspond to w_i, in the formula for concern.

[7]It may seem counterintuitive to assign greater weight to less serious effects (injury or illness) than to more serious ones. However, if there is much greater variability in less serious consequences (e.g., because serious ones hardly ever occur from any of the threats under consideration), then that attribute might deserve more attention.

Table 5-2 characterizes each of 5 possible threats to adolescents in terms of these 12 attributes. The values are taken from an elaborate test bed created to study prioritization processes at a hypothetical Centerville Middle School. The values were assigned to reflect circumstances that might be found in a typical U.S. school, and internally consistent, considering the specifics of this hypothetical school (i.e., size, location, age).[8] These values are represented by x_{ij} in the formula for concern. In the interests of simplicity, the utility assigned to each level of that attribute was set equal to the level, normalized to range from 0-1.0, across the five sources of vulnerability.

Combining attribute weights (w_i) with the estimates of outcomes (x_i) produces scores for overall concerns. Table 5-3 ranks the sources, from best (or least bad) to worst, for individuals with the four sets of values appearing in Table 5-3. For individuals focused on mortality (Set A), self-inflicted injury (i.e., suicide) draws the greatest concern and lead poisoning the least (in a school where lethal doses are impossible). If serious injury and illness also are important (Set B), then the less common infectious diseases at the school become the worst threat and the more common ones become more important. Giving weight to less serious injury and disease as well (Set C) further increases concern over common infectious diseases, and reduces that over intentional injury (whose nonfatal consequences at Centerville are rare). When weight is assigned to the qualitative attributes (rows 9–12 in Table 5-1), common infectious diseases drop in importance. They are understood very well, have immediate effects, and afford some measure of controllability (e.g., vaccination). As a result, they evoke little of the dread and discomfort associated with the less common infectious diseases or self-inflicted injury.

Thus, under the circumstances of this hypothetical school, relative concern over some of these sources of vulnerability varies considerably, depending on the weight given to the different attributes. On the other hand, lead poisoning merits relatively little concern, whatever the weighting scheme. Although its consequences can be terrible, in this (relatively new) school they are not that much of an issue. Lead poisoning might rank much higher in priorities set at an aging, urban school or in national priori-

---

[8]The project description is at: http://www.epp.cmu.edu/research/risk_ranking.html. Summary sheets describing the risks can be found at: http://www.epp.cmu.edu/research/risk-summary-sheets/risk1.html.

TABLE 5-2 Estimates of the Performance of 5 Sources of Adolescent Vulnerability on 12 Attributes

	Sources of Vulnerability				
Attribute	Common Infectious Diseases	Intentional Harm	Lead Poisoning	Less Common Infectious Diseases	Self-Inflicted Harm
Number of deaths per year	0.067	0.233	0	1	1
Chance in a million of death per year for the average student	0.071	0.286	0	1	1
Chance in a million of death per year for the student at highest risk	0.008	0.333	0	0.117	1
Greatest number of deaths in a single episode	0.04	0.107	0	1	0.107
More serious long-term injuries or illnesses (cases per year)	0.0005	0.01	0	1	0.02
Less serious long-term injuries or illnesses (cases per year)	0.2	0.05	1	0.2	0.3
More serious short-term injuries or illnesses (cases per year)	1	0.075	0	1	0.25
Less serious short-term injuries or illnesses (cases per year)	1	0.006	0	0.010	0.001
Time between exposure and health effects	0.5	1	0	0.5	1
Quality of scientific understanding	0	0.5	0	0	0.5
Uncertainty regarding death, illness, and injury	0.318	0.636	1	0.318	0.409
Ability of student/parent to control exposure	0.5	0	1	0.5	0

TABLE 5-3 Risk Rankings of 5 Sources of Adolescent Vulnerability Given Sets of Weights on 1 Set of 12 Attributes and Estimates from a Hypothetical Middle School

Rank		Set of Weights A	B	C	D
Best	1.	Lead poisoning	Lead poisoning	Intentional injury	Common infectious disease
	2.	Common infectious disease	Intentional injury	Lead poisoning	Lead poisoning
	3.	Intentional injury	Common infectious disease	Self-inflicted injury	Intentional injury
	4.	Less common infectious disease	Self-inflicted injury	Common infectious disease	Self-inflicted injury
Worst	5.	Self-inflicted injury	Less common infectious disease	Less common infectious disease	Less common infectious disease

ties that considered such schools. In that case, Centerville Middle School might have a mandate, and perhaps resources, to deal with a problem of relatively little local concern.

REFERENCES

Bendor, J. (1995). A model of muddling through. *American Political Science Review, 89,* 819-840.

Bentkover, J. D., Covello, V. T., & Mumpower, J. (Eds.). (1985). *Benefits assessment: The state of the art*. Dordrecht, The Netherlands: D. Reidel.

Breyer, S. (1993). *Breaking the vicious circle: Toward effective regulation.* Cambridge, MA: Harvard University Press.

Budescu, D. F., & Wallsten, T. S. (1995). Processing linguistic probabilities: General principles and empirical evidence. In J. R. Busemeyer, R. Hastie, & D. L. Medin (Eds.), *Decision making from a cognitive perspective* (pp. 275-318). New York: Academic Press.

Bureau of Labor Statistics. (1998). *NLS1997 handbook.* Washington, DC: U.S. Department of Labor.

Carnegie Mellon University. (2001). *Engineering and public policy risk analysis and risk communication.* Available: >http://www.epp.cmu.edu/research/EPP_risk.html>. [August 31, 2001].

Cohen, B., & Lee, I. S. (1979). A catalog of risks. *Health Physics, 36,* 707-722.

Crouch, E. A. C., & Wilson, R. (1981). *Risk-benefit analysis.* Boston: Ballinger.

Davies, J. C. (Ed.). (1996). *Comparing environmental risks.* Washington, DC: Resources for the Future.

Dawes, R. M. (1979). The robust beauty of improper linear models. *American Psychologist, 34,* 571-582.

Dawes, R. M., & Hastie, R. (in press). *Rational choice in an uncertain world* (2nd ed.). San Diego: Harcourt Brace.

Department of Health and Human Services. (2000). *Healthy people 2010.* Washington, DC: Author.

Federal Interagency Forum on Child and Family Statistics. (1997). *America's children: Key national indicators of well-being.* Washington, DC: Author.

Fischhoff, B. (1995). Ranking risks. *Risk: Health Safety & Environment, 6,* 189-200.

Fischhoff, B. (1999). Why (cancer) risk communication can be hard. *Journal of the National Cancer Institute Monographs, 25,* 7-13.

Fischhoff, B. (2000). Need to know: Analytical and psychological criteria. *Roger Williams University Law Review, 6,* 55-79.

Fischhoff, B., Bostrom, A., & Quadrel, M. J. (1997). Risk perception and communication. In R. Detels, J. McEwen, & G. Omenn (Eds.), *Oxford textbook of public health* (pp. 987-1002). London: Oxford University Press.

Fischhoff, B., Downs, J., & Bruine de Bruin, W. (1998). Adolescent vulnerability: A framework for behavioral interventions. *Applied and Preventive Psychology, 7,* 77-94.

Fischhoff, B., Lichtenstein, S., Slovic, P., Derby, S. L., & Keeney, R. L. (1981). *Acceptable risk.* New York: Cambridge University Press.

Fischhoff, B., Parker, A., Bruine de Bruin, W., Downs, J., Palmgren, C., Dawes, R.M., & Manski, C. (2000). Teen expectations for significant life events. *Public Opinion Quarterly, 64,* 189-205.

Fischhoff, B., Slovic, P., Lichtenstein, S., Read, S., & Combs, B. (1978). How safe is safe enough? A psychometric study of attitudes towards technological risks and benefits. *Policy Sciences, 8,* 127-152.

Fischhoff, B., Watson, S., & Hope, C. (1984). Defining risk. *Policy Sciences, 17,* 123-139.

Florig, H. K., Morgan, M. G., Morgan, K. M., Jenni, K. E., Fischhoff, B., Fischbeck, P. S., & DeKay, M. (in press). A test bed for studies of risk ranking. *Risk Analysis.*

Institute of Medicine. (1998). *Scientific opportunities and public needs: Improving priority setting and public input at the National Institutes of Health.* Committee on the NIH Research Priority-Setting Process. Health Sciences Section. Washington, DC: National Academy Press.

Institute of Medicine. (1999). *Toward environmental justice: Research, education, and health policy needs.* Committee on Environmental Justice. Health Sciences Section. Washington, DC: National Academy Press.

Jenni, K. (1997). *Attributes for risk evaluation.* Unpublished doctoral dissertation. Department of Engineering & Public Policy, Carnegie Mellon University.

Jessor, R., Donovan, J. E., & Costa, F. M. (1991). *Beyond adolescence.* New York, NY: Cambridge University Press.

Kahneman, D., Slovic, P., & Tversky, A. (Eds.). (1982). *Judgment under uncertainty: Heuristics and biases.* New York: Cambridge University Press.

Kahneman, D., & Tversky, A. (1979). Prospect theory: An analysis of decision under risk. *Econometrica, 47,* 263-281.

Keeney, R. L., & Raiffa, H. (1976). *Decisions with multiple objectives: Preferences and value tradeoffs.* New York: John Wiley.

Kolata, G. (2001, April 8). Putting a price tag on the priceless. *New York Times,* Section 4, p. 4.

Kubey, R., Larson, R., & Csikszentmihalyi, M. (1996). Experience sampling method applications to communications research. *Journal of Communication, 46*(2), 99-120.

Lerner, R. M. (in press). *Adolescence: Development, diversity, context, and application.* Upper Saddle River, NJ: Prentice-Hall.

Lichtenstein, S., Slovic, P., Fischhoff, B., Layman, M., & Combs, B. (1978). Judged frequency of lethal events. *Journal of Experimental Psychology: Human Learning and Memory, 4,* 551-578.

Lindblom, C. (1959). The science of muddling through. *Public Administration Review,* 79-88.

Loewenstein, G. (1996). Out of control: Visceral influences on decision making. *Organizational Behavior and Human Decision Processes, 65,* 272-292.

Long, J., & Fischhoff, B. (2000). Setting risk priorities: A formal model. *Risk Analysis, 20,* 339-351.

Lowrance, W. (1975). *Of acceptable risk.* San Francisco: Freeman.

Masten, A. S. (2001). Ordinary magic: Resilience processes in development. *American Psychologist, 56,* 227-238.

McFadden, D. (1999). Rationality for economists? *Journal of Risk and Uncertainty, 19,* 73-105.

Macintyre, S., & West, P. (1993). What does the phrase "safer sex" mean to you? Understanding among Glaswegian 18 year olds in 1990. *AIDS, 7,* 121-126.

Morgan, K. M., DeKay, M. L., Fischbeck, P. S., Morgan, M. G., Fischhoff, B., & Florig, H. K. (in press). A deliberative method for ranking risks: Evaluating validity and usefulness. *Risk Analysis.*

Morgan, M. G., Fischhoff, B., Bostrom, A., & Atman, C. (2001). *Risk communication: The mental models approach.* New York: Cambridge University Press.

Morgan, M. G., Fischhoff, B., Lave, L., & Fischbeck, P. (1996). A proposal for ranking risks within federal agencies. In C. Davies (Ed.), *Comparing environmental risks* (pp. 111-147). Washington, DC: Resources for the Future.

National Institutes of Health. (1998). *Setting research priorities at the National Institutes of Health.* Washington, DC: Author.

National Research Council. (1983). *Risk assessment in the federal government: Managing the process.* Committee on the Institutional Means for Assessment of Risks to Public Health. Commission on Life Sciences. Washington, DC: National Academy Press.

National Research Council. (1996). *Understanding risk: Informing decisions in a democratic society.* Committee on Risk Characterization. P. C. Stern & H. V. Fineberg (Eds.). Commission on Behavioral and Social Sciences and Education. Washington, DC: National Academy Press.

Office of Technology Assessment. (1995). *Risks to students in school* (OTA-ENV-633). Washington, DC: U.S. Congress. Available: <http://www.ota.nap.edu/pubs.html>. [August 8, 2001].

Quadrel, M. J., Fischhoff, B., & Davis, W. (1993). Adolescent (in)vulnerability. *American Psychologist, 48,* 102-116.

Schriver, K. A. (1989). Evaluating text quality: The continuum from text-focused to reader-focused methods. *IEEE Transactions on Professional Communication, 32,* 238-255.

Schwarz, N. (1999). Self reports. *American Psychologist, 54,* 93-105.

Simon, H. A. (1957). *Models of man.* Cambridge, MA: MIT Press.

Slovic, P. (1987). Perceptions of risk. *Science, 236,* 280-285.

Starr, C. (1969). Social benefit versus technological risk. *Science, 165,* 1232-1238.

Tengs, T. O., Adams, M. E., Pliskin, J. S., Safran, D. G., Siegel, J. E., Weinstein, M. C., & Graham, J. D. (1995). 500 lifesaving interventions and their cost-effectiveness. *Risk Analysis, 15,* 369-390.

Tengs, T. O., & Wallace, A. (2000). One thousand quality of life estimates. *Medical Care, 36,* 583-637.

United Nations. (1989). *Convention on the rights of the child.* New York: Author.

vonWinterfeldt, D., & Edwards, W. (1986). *Decision analysis and behavioral research.* New York: Cambridge University Press.

Weinstein, N. D. (1987). Unrealistic optimism about susceptibility to health problems. *Journal of Behavioral Medicine, 19,* 481-500.

Appendix

Workshop Materials

Agenda
March 13, 2001

8:15 a.m.–8:45 a.m.
Registration and Continental Breakfast

8:45 a.m.–9:00 a.m.
Welcome, Introductions, and Purpose of the Workshop

Elena O. Nightingale, Workshop Co-Chair, Scholar-in Residence, National Academy of Sciences
Baruch Fischhoff, Workshop Co-Chair. University Professor, Department of Social and Decision Sciences, Department of Engineering and Public Policy, Carnegie Mellon University

9:00 a.m.–10:15 a.m.
Threats to Adolescent Well-Being: A Conceptual Framework

Robert William Blum, Professor, Department of Pediatrics, University of Minnesota
(co-authors: Clea S. McNeely and James Nonnemaker)
Reactors/Discussants:
Lloyd Kolbe, Director, Division of Adolescent and School Health, Centers for Disease Control and Prevention
Beatrix A. Hamburg, Visiting Scholar, Department of Psychiatry, Cornell University Medical College

Q&A and General Discussion

- What do we know about vulnerability?
- What factors predispose adolescents to risk?
- What vulnerabilities do adolescents with special needs face?
- What buffers exist to reduce risk?
- What do recent studies tell us about trends that are associated with poor outcomes?
- What role(s) does the environment play in vulnerability?
- What opportunities exist for promoting adolescent well-being?
- What are the consequences of failure to support adolescent well-being?
- Can a new conceptual model help us to understand and moderate adolescent vulnerability?

10:15 a.m.–10:30 a.m.
Break

10:30 a.m.–11:45 a.m.
Modeling the Payoffs of Interventions to Reduce Adolescent Vulnerability

Martha R. Burt, Program Director and Principal Research Associate, Urban Institute (co-authors: Janine M. Zweig and John Roman)
Reactors/Discussants:
*Susan P. Curnan, Associate Professor and Chair, MM/MBA Program in Child, Youth, and Family Studies and Director, Center for Youth and Communities, Heller Graduate School, Brandeis University
Peter Edelman, Professor of Law, Georgetown University Law Center

Q&A and General Discussion

- How can social cost be defined?
- What models help us understand lifelong costs and benefits of risky behaviors in adolescence?

---

*Note: Ms. Curnan responded in writing as she was prevented from traveling by weather.

- Why should society be motivated to address the problems experienced by adolescents?
- What can we learn about adolescent vulnerability if we view adolescents as individuals, human capital, or a societal value?
- What is the cost of adolescents' high-risk behavior to society relative to other societal costs?
- What impact can interventions and public investments have on reducing adolescent vulnerability?

11:45 a.m.–12:30 p.m.
Quick Lunch

12:30 p.m.–1:45 p.m.
Adolescent Vulnerability: Measurement and Priority Setting

Baruch Fischhoff, Professor, Carnegie Mellon University (co-author: Henry Willis)
Reactors/Discussants:
Matthew Stagner, Principal Research Associate, Population Studies Center, Urban Institute
Mark Cohen, Associate Professor, Owen Graduate School of Management, Vanderbilt University

Q&A and General Discussion

- What approaches can be taken to assess the burden of vulnerability?
- What are the components of the full burden of vulnerability?
- What alternative ways can be used to measure and weight risks?
- What indices are useful to monitor progress in reducing vulnerability?
- What values govern funding priorities and mechanisms?
- What social mechanisms can be used to set priorities to reduce adolescent vulnerabilities?

1:45 p.m.–3:00 p.m.
Perceptions of Risk and Vulnerability

Susan G. Millstein, Professor of Pediatrics, Division of Adolescent Medicine, University of California at San Francisco (co-author: Bonnie Halpern-Felsher)
Reactors/Discussants:
Richard M. Lerner, Bergstrom Chair in Applied Developmental Science, Eliot-Pearson Department of Child Development, Tufts University
Ann Masten, Professor, Institute of Child Development, University of Minnesota

Q&A and General Discussion

- What data illuminate our knowledge about adolescents' beliefs about risk and vulnerability?
- What data illuminate our knowledge about adults' beliefs about adolescents' risk and vulnerability?
- How do beliefs about risks influence judgments about risk taking?
- What do we know about adolescents' abilities to manage risk and opportunity?
- How accurate are adolescents' and adults' perceptions of risk? How do they compare? What are the important sources of bias in their perceptions?

3:00 p.m.–3:15 p.m.
Break

3:15 p.m.–4:30 p.m.
Opportunities for Bridging Research, Policy, and Practice

Heather Weiss, Harvard Family Research Project, Harvard University
Gary Melton, Director, Institute on Family and Neighborhood Life, Clemson University
Shepherd Smith, President, Institute for Youth Development

Q&A and General Discussion

4:30 p.m.
Concluding Remarks and Adjourn

Baruch Fischhoff and Elena O, Nightingale

PRESENTERS

Robert William Blum, Center for Adolescent Health, University of Minnesota-Twin Cities
Martha R. Burt, Urban Institute, Washington, DC
Mark Cohen, Owen Graduate School of Management, Vanderbilt University
*Susan P. Curnan, Heller Graduate School, Brandeis University
Peter Edelman, Law Center, Georgetown University
Baruch Fischhoff, Department of Social and Decision Sciences, Carnegie Mellon University
Beatrix A. Hamburg, Psychiatry Department, Cornell University Medical College
Lloyd J. Kolbe, Division of Adolescent and School Health, Centers for Disease Control and Prevention, Atlanta, GA
Richard M. Lerner, Eliot-Pearson Department of Child Development, Tufts University
Ann S. Masten, Institute of Child Development, University of Minnesota-Twin Cities
Clea McNeely, Division of General Pediatrics and Adolescent Health, University of Minnesota-Twin Cities
Gary B. Melton, Institute on Family and Neighborhood Life, Clemson University
Susan G. Millstein, Division of Adolescent Medicine, University of California-San Francisco
Elena O. Nightingale, Board on Children, Youth, and Families, National Research Council, Washington, DC

---

*Note: Ms. Curnan responded in writing as she was prevented from traveling by weather.

Shepherd Smith, The Institute for Youth Development, Washington, DC
Matthew Stagner, Population Studies Center, Urban Institute, Washington, DC
Heather Weiss, Harvard Family Research Project, Harvard University

PARTICIPANTS

Cheryl Alexander, Department of Population and Family Health Services, Center for Adolescent Health, Johns Hopkins School of Hygiene and Public Health
Nan Marie Astone, School of Hygiene and Public Health, The Johns Hopkins University
Stephani Becker, Lucile Packard Foundation for Children's Health, Palo Alto, CA
Jennifer L. Brooks, Child Trends, Washington, DC
Brett Brown, Social Indicators Research, Child Trends, Washington, DC
Sarah Brown, National Campaign to Prevent Teen Pregnancy, Washington, DC
Barney Cohen, Committee on Population, National Research Council
Nancy Crowell, Committee on Law and Justice, National Research Council
Marilyn Dabady, Youth Population and Military Recruitment, Board on Behavioral, Cognitive, and Sensory Sciences, National Research Council
Paula Duncan, Vermont Agency of Human Services
Valerie Durrant, Committee on Population, National Research Council
Glen Elliott, Langley Porter Psychiatric Institute, University of California-San Francisco
Ellen Fern, National Partnerships and State and Local Action, National Campaign to Prevent Teen Pregnancy, Washington, DC
Bridget Freeman, Healthy Adolescent Project, American Psychological Association, Washington, DC
Beth Frerking, Casey Journalism Center on Children and Families, College Park, MD
Jennifer Gootman, Board on Children, Youth, and Families, National Research Council and Institute of Medicine
Sandra Graham, Department of Education, University of California-Los Angeles
Robert C. Granger, William T. Grant Foundation, New York, NY

Erica Greenstein, National Campaign to Prevent Teen Pregnancy, Washington, DC
Ruth Toby Gross, Department of Pediatrics, Stanford University
Umit Guvenc, Department of Engineering and Public Policy, Carnegie Mellon University
Elizabeth C. Hair, Child Trends, Washington, DC
Bonnie Halpern-Felsher, Division of Adolescent Medicine, University of California-San Francisco
Isadora R. Hare, Office on Adolescent Health, U.S. Department of Health and Human Services, Rockville, MD
Jamie Davis Hueston, Indian Health Service, U.S. Department of Health and Human Services, Rockville, MD
Renee R. Jenkins, Department of Pediatrics and Child Health, College of Medicine, Howard University
Meredith Kelsey, Office of Planning and Evaluation, U.S. Department of Health and Human Services, Washington, DC
Michele Kipke, Board on Children, Youth, and Families, National Research Council and Institute of Medicine
Laura Lippman, National Center for Education Statistics, Washington, DC
Andrea MacKay, Office of Analysis, Epidemiology, and Health Promotion, National Center for Health Statistics, Centers for Disease Control and Prevention, Hyattsville, MD
Jeffrey Merrill, Robert Wood Johnson Medical School, Piscataway, NJ
Laura E. Montgomery, Federal Interagency Forum on Child and Family Statistics, National Center for Health Statistics, Centers for Disease Control and Prevention, Hyattsville, MD
Susan Newcomer, National Institute for Child Health and Human Development, Bethesda, MD
James Nonnemaker, Division of General Pediatrics and Adolescent Health, University of Minnesota-Twin Citites
Catherine Pino, Carnegie Corporation of New York
Holly Reed, Committee on Population, National Research Council
John Roman, Urban Institute, Washington, DC
Patrick Rooney, National Center for Education Statistics, Washington, DC
Jane Ross, Center for Social and Economic Studies, National Research Council

Donna E. Shalala, Washington, DC
Andrea Solarz, American Psychological Association, Washington, DC
Laura Sessions Stepp, Style Section, *The Washington Post*, Washington, DC
Elizabeth Sullivan, Development and Finance Assistant, National Campaign to Prevent Teen Pregnancy, Washington, DC
Rochelle Tafolla, Media Program Associate, National Campaign to Prevent Teen Pregnancy, Washington, DC
Ruby Takanishi, Foundation for Child Development, New York, NY
Bill Treanor, Youth Today, Washington, DC
Sharon Vandivere, Child Trends, Washington, DC
Patience H. White, Pediatric Rheumatology, Children's National Medical Center, Bethesda, MD
Jennifer Widness, Youth Leadership Team, National Campaign to Prevent Teen Pregnancy, Washington, DC
Henry Willis, Department of Engineering and Public Policy, Carnegie Mellon University
Audrey Yowell, Office of Adolescent Health, Maternal and Child Health Bureau, U.S. Department of Health and Human Services, Rockville, MD
Jonathan F. Zaff, Child Trends, Washington, DC
Diana Zuckerman, National Center for Policy Research for Women and Families, Washington, DC
Janine Zweig, Labor and Social Policy Center, Urban Institute, Washington, DC